On Mothering Multiples

On Mothering Multiples
Complexities and Possibilities

edited by
Kathy Mantas

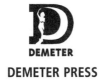

DEMETER

DEMETER PRESS

Funded by the Government of Canada
Financé par la gouvernement du Canada | Canadä

Demeter Press
140 Holland Street West
P. O. Box 13022
Bradford, ON L3Z 2Y5
Tel: (905) 775-9089
Email: info@demeterpress.org
Website: www.demeterpress.org

Demeter Press logo based on the sculpture "Demeter" by Maria-Luise Bodirsky
<www.keramik-atelier.bodirsky.de>

Printed and Bound in Canada

Front cover artwork: Mangalika Sriyani Meewalaarachchi, "The endless spring of love," 2015, oil pastel drawing, 11.8 inches x 13.8 inches.

Library and Archives Canada Cataloguing in Publication
    On mothering multiples : complexities and possibilities / edited by Kathy Mantas.

Includes bibliographical references.
ISBN 978-1-926452-78-4 (paperback)

    1. Motherhood. 2. Mothers. 3. Multiple birth. 4. Multiple pregnancy.
5. Childbirth. 6. Conception. I. Mantas, Kathy, 1966-, author, editor

HQ759.O53 2016   306.874'3   C2016-900333-7

To my daughter Seraphina Helana,
without whom this book would not have been written.

In memory of
my son Angelo Emmanuel

Similarly, in commemoration of all multiples
who were/are with us for a short while
but who are with us always in our hearts.

Table of Contents

Acknowledgements

I am most appreciative of all the authors gathered on these pages who have contributed their provocative and evocative stories and essays with honesty and grace. I thank you for your patience, generosity, and insights. Your stories inspire and give me courage. It was a real honour to write and partake in this collection with you.

I would like to acknowledge Lynda P. Haddon and Bonnie L. Schultz for their bountiful foreword to this edited collection. I thank you for the many years of wisdom that you bring to this collection.

I would like to thank Mangalika Sriyani Meewalaarachchi for her hard work on the cover image of this book and for making mothering the subject of her art.

Within the organization of Demeter Press, I would like to thank Angie Deveau for her help with the early stages of the books conception (e.g., the call for papers). Similarly, I would like to express my sincere thanks to Andrea O'Reilly, publisher of Demeter Press, who from the beginning supported the creation of this book with patience, understanding, flexibility, and persistent nudges of encouragement and support. Likewise, I would like to thank Jesse O'Reilly-Conlin, the copy editor, for his assistance with the publication process.

I also give thanks to Lori Ann Manis, my proofreader, for her careful attention to MLA details and thoughtful approach to the editing process. It would have been impossible to meet the editing deadlines, in the middle and end stages of this process, without her ongoing support and expertise. Thank you!

My gratitude also extends to the editors of *Performing Motherhood: Artistic, Activist, and Everyday Enactments*—especially Amber E. Kinser and Terri Hawkes—and, the editor of *Intensive Mothering: The Cultural Contradictions of Modern Motherhood*, Linda Rose Ennis, for sharing their wisdom and knowledge of the editing process with generosity, and their words of support.

My thanks also go to the tour guides and Kimberley Lyon, museum director of *The Quints Museum,* for being so giving of their time and their willingness to share their expertise with me this past July 2015. I also thank Patti Carr, museum director of North Bay and District Chamber of Commerce, for proofing and approving the final draft of my closing and for sharing with me the two photographs of the Dionne quintuplets, as infants and teenagers, found in the closing.

Additionally, I would like to thank Kimberley Weatherall—the former executive director of Multiple Births Canada (MBC)/ Naissances Multiple Canada, board member and past chair for the International Council of Multiple Birth Organizations (ICOMBO)—for introducing me to various multiple birth communities and her genuine interest in the book.

I also give thanks to the external reviewers for their time, support, and willingness to appraise this manuscript and offer thoughtful feedback.

Finally, I would like to extend my deep gratitude to my family; especially to my partner Roger, for his understanding and careful reading of my bookends (opening and closing) in the pre-external review phase of the process; my daughter Seraphina for keeping me grounded and feeding my muse; and my mother Pagona for her ongoing support and grandmothering as I worked, often into the night and through the weekends, to bring this edited collection to fruition.

For all this, I feel a deep sense of gratitude.

Foreword

LYNDA P. HADDON AND BONNIE L. SCHULTZ

REFLECTIONS ON MOTHERING take on a unique hue when the prospect of "multiples" comes into play. At once, multiple lives emerge from a single pregnancy and the group process that follows provides a fascinating perspective on what it means to mother. Indeed, the possibilities, challenges, joys, and demands are themselves multiple in the multiple births scenario.

While fertility treatments have increased the likelihood that pregnancies will result in two, three, or more babies, both our twin pregnancies occurred spontaneously. Our era was prior to the introduction of modern day reproductive advances and before anyone would intrusively ask whether conception was "natural or not." For those not a part of the multiple birth culture of parenting twins or other higher order multiples, it has always been a challenge to fully understand our lives; this was certainly true of our personal experiences. Multiples were a delightful oddity that drew mainly superficial attention. The true challenges were hidden from view. It is no wonder that we were drawn to peers for collective support, and we clearly recognized that our group did not necessarily include parents of singleton births, no matter how large the family. Furthermore, prenatal classes for singletons were helpful but only to a point.

In the 1980s, community resources aimed at the challenges of multiple birth families were meagre and often non-existent in many communities. Moreover, misunderstandings and cultural stereotypes were legion. What went unrecognized was the complexity for the mother, babies, and family constellation. Everything from the mechanics of breastfeeding two or more unique infants to supporting couples and family life under the stress of caring for two or more infants concurrently was barely, if ever, discussed. The false presumption of the time was that any prenatal or postnatal class would suffice, and the parent should simply multiply by two or three, as the situation demanded. Monozygotic (identical twins) babies were, more often than not, dressed identically, and the identity needs of such children went unrecognized.

The situation called out for change. Parents raising twins, triplets, and more comprised a unique set that faced very different challenges that needed to be understood in their own terms. Mothering, in particular, had to be reimagined to understand how women faced with this situation coped and viewed the experience. The unique context of multiple births begins with the bodily sensations felt *in utero*: two or more growing lives are sharing one body. This one-for-two ratio (or even one-for-three or more) remains the core of the maternal experience throughout the children's development. The ratio creates complex opportunities for sharing, choosing, relating, loving, and even conflict management that reflect unique pressure points and challenges. Nurturing two or more children simultaneously is never easy nor is creating a life space that must be shared, as the womb was once shared, and that must allow the children to develop strong, individual and self-affirming identities.

Another complex yet often overlooked factor that is frequently a key part of the multiple births context is the relationship between multiples and their singleton siblings. This dynamic deserves mentioning in large part because it takes sensitivity and skill to cope with and can be a preoccupying factor for both parents and singleton siblings alike.

The "miracle" of spontaneous multiple births still happens with the rarity it always did. Life creating, however, has been transformed by reproductive technologies. Had it not been for advances in these technologies, mothering multiples would have likely remained a more extraordinary event. What was once perceived as simply a matter of chance is now a sign of the growing co-operation between human reproduction and medical science. Yet it remains to be seen how this close and growing collaboration affects how women understand and relate to their bodies and view the pregnancy experience itself. Furthermore, such reproductive advances have created a new class of offspring: children of assisted reproduction. These children are highly prized, and they reflect the successful outcome of the partnership between the conceiving woman or couple and the medical industry. Again, questions abound as to whether these children are viewed differently as a result of their origins or whether their origins are mainly irrelevant. In turn, we could ponder how this might affect how such children see themselves.

As a result of supporting bereaved multiple birth parents, grandparents and surviving co-multiples over the past twenty-six years, Lynda has also experienced first-hand the underbelly of this explosive growth in assisted reproduction. Indeed, advancements in technology, particularly in vitro fertilization, have led to not only more babies and more multiples but also more losses. The enhanced probability of multiple births also raises the risk of loss. This loss can include the loss of a fetus in utero through natural causes or fetus reduction by the same medical professionals who implanted the fertilized ova in willing women eager to be mothers. In addition, there is the inherent difficulty of mourning vanishing twins whose only existence arises in early ultrasounds. In other words, the experience of loss in multiple births can be as unique and challenging as any other part of this complex experience. Indeed, there is a community of mothers, some raising surviving co-multiples, who grieve for their deceased babies for a lifetime as well as for the surviving co-multiples themselves who live a life of identity incompleteness, as if they were missing a part of themselves. Hence, bereavement support is a fundamental service to the community of multiple birth parents in a way that has no parallel in the singleton context. It is a testament to the need for people to mourn their losses, even when these losses occurred before, at, or sometime after birth.

In popular culture, multiple births are viewed as an opportunity for "double joy." The general perception is that two children for the price of one is a deal most mothers-to-be would not turn down. Nonetheless, little attention has been given to the fact that there is no guarantee both babies, or higher order multiples, will receive the same biological benefit in utero. Nature is not necessarily known for its fairness. Such differences in what each baby receives nutritionally in utero can lead to significantly different outcomes for the children—one with special needs, for example, and one without. Besides the emotional complexity for the twins themselves, parenting in this situation can be difficult. This complexity illustrates another dimension of parenting in multiple births that has no specific parallel in the singleton situation.

One of the most fascinating aspects of the multiple experience, at least as recounted by multiples themselves, concerns the depth of connection that they can feel with each other. This closeness highlights the potential distinction between being a sibling in general and being a twin or triplet sibling. Much has been written by children of multiple births who, in the form of personal narratives or testimonies, document the uncanny sense of connection and communication between them that defies logical explanation. The underlying premise appears to be that twins and other higher order multiples who share an intimacy in utero benefit from a unique connection that links them in ways unmatched by other family relations. Mythical or not, twins or higher order multiples can project the image that they are less alone in the universe than the rest of us. On the other hand, monozygotic twins can also argue that they must bear the fate of not being as unique as singletons. Of course, as a partial compensation, these one-egg multiples remain the darlings of geneticists, which adds to their allure.

This fascination brings to mind that twins and triplets as infants and young children are often a focus of attention precisely because they are multiples. It is not a status earned, however, and the repercussions are mixed. Naturally, it is nice to be noticed but at the same time it works against the need for individuation of identity. Being a twin or triplet does not preclude the necessity to develop one's own identity, which can weigh on the parent when the community appears more interested in the children's multiple status than the unique personality of each child. Nowadays, one hears much less reference to "the twins" than was commonplace in past eras.

Today, much more is available to mothers and couples facing the birth of twins, triplets, and more than when we gave birth and entered this community. Multiple birth organizations offer vital information, support, and the kinds of preplanning that really make a difference when the babies arrive. Nonetheless, multiple births are still the whirlwind that they always were and remain a major life adjustment for all parents, grandparents, and guardians alike. As in many areas, however, knowledge is power, and conveying the right information or support at the time that it is needed can make a difference and contribute significantly to the health and well-being of children and families. In our view, the evolution of self-help organizations dedicated to multiple births in the past thirty years or more has been instrumental to improving the experience for children, parents, and families. On the other hand, government and industry policies regarding parental leave can still miss the mark and fail to make a place for the specific demands and needs of this community. For instance, there is often no recognition that having two or more babies born simultaneously could require the work leave of two parents, each worthy of government tax subsidy or support. As much as psychological research stresses the vital importance of infant care, public policy can still ignore the special context and enhanced demands faced by parents of multiple births.

The multiple births experience, in its unique and sometimes daunting complexity, awaits literature that reflects the *realpolitik* of maternal care in the face of evolving social and reproductive realities. Thankfully, this important book makes a significant start in this direction. The reductionist tendency for self-help to be equated with how-to manuals has probably added to the problem of oversimplification and omission, particularly with respect to the realities of the multiple births experience. Of course, many of these experiences are positive, self-affirming, and fulfilling, but we should also not ignore that multiple births include increased risks for prematurity, loss, and disability, especially in higher order multiples. It is a key strength that this book confronts the difficult, the mythical, and the complex, often through the lens of its contributors' personal experiences. To be sure, what is needed are more works that help prospective parents, health professionals, and social scientists enter the world of multiples, because this world also intersects with key societal issues such as infertility, reproductive technologies and their impact on infant health, maternal essentialism, breastfeeding, politics of childcare, and the changing perspectives on the notion of family beyond normative lines. The reader is treated in these pages to just such an endeavour, a book interwoven with personal and artistic narratives that share the joys, sorrows, risks, fears, and wonderment of conceiving, bearing, and raising twins, triplets, or more. As such, self-help emerges from its common prosaic roots in these pages to resemble a form of witnessing, reflecting, examining, and expressing that comes much closer to capturing what is essential about this amazing mothering experience.

Opening

KATHY MANTAS

ALTHOUGH THIS BOOK was inspired in part by my own story, its current form was birthed one fall afternoon when my life was disrupted, and I was confined to my home. I found myself, unwillingly in the beginning, forced to slow down. This event, which involved rest, in time created a space for indwelling and helped me to transform an unanticipated interruption into a pause that was filled with possibility. One can say that I had an encounter with a Muse—the one within me, within all of us. As Mary Daly states, "My Muse or Muses invariably waited until evening to arrive and stayed around until I was more than ready to collapse with fatigue" (xix-xx) or, in my case, until I was house-bound after my surgery. This idea of an edited collection on the topic of mothering multiples stayed with me in the weeks and months that followed, and over time, this interruption turned into a pregnant pause and led to the conception of an idea that eventually took the shape of an anthology. This book is a labour of love.

This is not a book about "how to" or "what to do when" or "tips and guidelines," nor is it a "step-by-step" manual or "program" to follow; it is neither a "guidebook," nor a "handbook"; and it is certainly not an "everything you wanted or needed to know about mothering multiples" book. Instead, it is a book of musings—examinations, considerations, speculations, dwellings on, contemplations, ponderings, reflections, explorations, ruminations, revisits, and reveries—on the topic of mothering multiples. These essays, both creative and scholarly, are meant to bemuse and amuse, provoke and evoke, bring insight and inform, inspire and haunt, disturb and challenge, and invoke and raise questions.

This edited collection also celebrates the fullness of the experience of mothering multiples at all its stages—from infertility to fertility, from preconception to conception, post-birth and beyond—and in all its forms. It commemorates all the little lives who take this journey—at all phases of life—as a twin, triplet, or other higher order multiple and all those who mother them. As Michelle Walks and Naomi McPherson state in their edited collection *An Anthology of Mothering* mothering "is not simply about an institution (of motherhood), nor a biological or social role (a mother), but about engaging acts of *mothering*, regardless of institutional involvement, biology, sex, and gender ... *mothering* occurs whether or not it is biologically, legally, and/or socially/culturally recognized as such" (x).

By weaving together scholarly, creative, and blended forms, written by a diverse group of authors, a "polyvalent [text] ... used to *vivify* interpretation" (Lather 91) is created.

My hope is that this form—which creates openings for the often silenced, neglected and marginalized voices and stories to emerge and be heard (mothering multiples with special needs, prematurity, infertility and assisted reproductive technologies (ART), queer narratives of infertility and ART procedures in relationship to multiples, loss and multiples, breastfeeding, childcare, to name a few)—will contribute to filling some of the gaps in our experience and in the literature as well as extend understandings of the experience of mothering multiples in all its complexities. Furthermore, specifically within the context and experience of multiples, this book also acknowledges that mothering multiples means multiple realities simultaneously experienced.

As the editor of this collection, I was faced with the responsibility of presenting these essays, scholarly and creative in nature, in a way that is both respectful of and sensitive to the authors who so generously shared their stories. I hope that I have succeeded in this task. Like multiples, these essays are *alike and not alike.* My life has been enriched through this edited collection, and I have been inspired by the words and images shared by all the contributing authors who have lovingly shared their experiences. It is really the contributors in this collection who are the experts here.

These essays, though connected, do not fit into fixed categories. My wish is that, taken as a whole, they will nurture understanding as well as bring an expanded awareness of the many viewpoints through which the topic of mothering multiples may be considered. Furthermore, my desire is that these chapters will offer not only musings inviting us to think more deeply on and about mothering multiples but also possibilities and hope. To this end, I invite you to enter this diverse gathering of texts and images and move through the pages in a way that resonates with you. This collection of work, which I have attempted to present in the most fluid way possible, allows you to move back and forth between scholarly essays, to take a visual pause when you encounter an interlude, and to linger longer when you happen to come upon a narrative. Perhaps in the process an image will emerge, a story will surface, a question will arise, or an encounter with your Muse will transpire, and you too will be invited to bring your own ruminations to this gathering.

Warmest regards,

Kathy Mantas

WORKS CITED

Daly, Mary. *Gyn/Ecology: The Metaethics of Radical Feminism.* Boston, MA: Beacon Press, 1978. Print.

Lather, Patti. *Getting Smart: Feminist Research and Pedagogy With/In the Postmodern.* New York: Routledge, 1991. Print.

Walks, Michelle, and Naomi McPherson, eds. *An Anthropology of Mothering.* Bradford, ON: Demeter Press, 2011. Print.

1.
"Why Should We Not Be Depressed?"

A Population at Risk, and Problems with Traditional Understandings of Multiple Motherhood

CHRISTIE E. BOLCH AND JANE R. FISHER

THE BIRTH OF AN INFANT is associated with a period of psychological adjustment that presents developmental challenges to all women, some of whom will go on to experience a period of sustained low mood and/or debilitating worry. When the birth is not of one infant but two or three or more, the challenge is not doubled or tripled as might be expected but is increased exponentially. The physical workload accompanying the birth of multiple children is difficult to appreciate unless experienced first-hand. The work of mothering is quite literally never finished, and there is always more than one child needing (or demanding) attention. A breastfeeding mother of newborn twins is likely to be giving sixteen to twenty-four feeds per day and changing twenty nappies (Gromada and Hurlburt 65). Fortunately, feeds decrease to thirteen per day at twenty weeks (Damato and Burant 742) but at all ages, basic care needs are increased. It takes 197 hours (out of a possible 168) per week to provide care for newborn triplets ("Having Twins and Triplets"). Once the infants become mobile, they move in opposite directions. Not only are demands increased but mothers of multiples also have diminished access to resources that safeguard their well-being, including opportunities to rest and recover and to pursue their own interests.

When attempting to describe some of the challenges facing mothers of multiples, there is a risk of painting an exceedingly bleak picture. In recent years, researchers have increasingly drawn attention to the considerable psychosocial risks associated with multiple birth (Bryan, "The Impact of Multiple Preterm Births"

24), in particular for mothers (Ellison and Hall 405; Fisher and Stocky 506). The challenges of the early months are considerably better documented than the longer-term implications. From the outset, we wish to state emphatically that despite the challenges, mothering multiples has many wonderful facets. We undertook an investigation of the quality of life of mothers of twins and triplets (average age 5 and a half years), which included a novel inventory of "multiple-specific" comments that mothers could endorse or reject (Bolch et al., "The MultiQOL Study," 418). Almost without exception, mothers strongly endorsed the "positive" items (e.g., "I feel a sense of achievement that I have raised my multiples to this point"; "I enjoy watching my multiples interact with each other"), indicating they could clearly identify the benefits. However, although these positive aspects were experienced and acknowledged, ultimately they made no measureable difference to the mothers' quality of life. The *less* positive aspects of mothering multiples, however—the unrelenting workload, constant demands on mothers' time and attention, and (for many) the experience of a difficult pregnancy and birth—were clearly and strongly associated with mothers' present and diminished quality of life. It is with these less comfortable aspects of mothering multiples that we are concerned.

REACTION TO LEARNING OF MULTIPLE GESTATION

For mothers conceiving multiples with assisted reproductive technologies (ART), the possibility of multiple birth will have probably been imagined before pregnancy. Mothers who elect transfer of two or more embryos during an in vitro fertilization (IVF) treatment cycle, or who take ovulation induction medication, are informed of the increased risk of multiple birth associated with such procedures. For most mothers of multiples, however, the diagnosis comes unexpectedly (Bryan, "Psychological Aspects" 827). Even mothers conceiving with ART may not necessarily have appreciated their risk of actually bearing multiples, since they considered dual embryo transfer as a means to increase probability of a *single* baby. Several authors have documented the range of responses to diagnosis of multiple pregnancy (Reinheckel et al. 55; Spillman 6; Bryan, "Psychological Aspects"). As Bryan wrote: "A diagnosis of a multiple pregnancy is always a surprise, often a shock, and may sometimes cause considerable distress" (827).

This range of responses contrasts with the prevailing discourse in anglophone and high-income countries that multiples are "cute," and a multiple pregnancy is something "special," which should be a cause for celebration rather than dismay. There is, in fact, a subset of fertile women trying to conceive who actively seek means of increasing the chance of a multiple pregnancy, and advice is available (Fierro "Top 10 Ways to Increase Your Chances of Having Twins"). Such women not infrequently post questions on multiple birth parenting online message boards, asking for advice. The following words from a mother of twins characterizes the usual response: "I think some of the women who ask these questions just want the attention multiples brings, but have no idea how much more work it is!" ("I Would Love to Have Twins").

For parents who have experienced infertility, the occurrence of multiple pregnancy may be perceived by others as providing them with an "instant family" (Baor and Blickstein 127). There is little opportunity for parents expecting multiples to acknowledge publicly, or even privately, any ambivalence that they may feel about the situation (Fisher, Rowe, and Hammarberg 1410). One mother described this on her parenting weblog: "My doctor and the nurses were all smiles as they congratulated me on the surprising news; meanwhile, I plastered on a fake smile because deep down, I was scared out of my mind" ("Are You Freaking Out").

EXPERIENCE OF A "HIGH-RISK" PREGNANCY

In medical terms, all multiple pregnancies are "high-risk" pregnancies. Risks include premature labour, high blood pressure, and severe morning sickness. However, many multiple pregnancies proceed without significant complications, resulting in the birth of healthy infants at term. The terminology of elevated risk, though accurate, is alarming to some women. Evidence is limited regarding the experiences of mothers whose multiple pregnancies are unremarkable, except for the fact that they *are* multiple.

Mothers undergoing medically complicated pregnancies are generally aware of their elevated risk (Gupton, Heaman, and

Cheung 192), and elevated risk has been shown to be associated with increased antenatal maternal anxiety (Stahl and Hundley 298). Mothers pregnant with multiples may be diverted to specialized high-risk obstetric clinics, and depending on circumstances, may be advised against particular birth practices such as vaginal birth, and will, almost certainly, be advised against vaginal birth without epidural anaesthesia (Vayssière et al. 12).

A qualitative study using focus groups with fourteen women attending a non-specific "high-risk" pregnancy clinic in the United Kingdom concluded that these mothers were reassured by greater medical involvement, including frequent monitoring (O'Brien, Quenby, and Lavender 82). However, these mothers were not representative of "high-risk" mothers in general, as each had previously experienced preterm birth and most had experienced perinatal loss. Multiple gestations were not reported. There are sound reasons for mothers who have previously experienced preterm birth and/or bereavement to welcome close monitoring; these may not apply equally to mothers of multiples, who usually do not have such a history.

One study investigated the impact of a medical diagnosis of "high-risk" pregnancy on mothers' psychological states on a group of German mothers who were designated "high risk" according to local obstetric guidelines but who would be considered "low risk" outside Germany (Stahl and Hundley 298). Factors in this context which led to a "high risk" label included age (<18 years or >35 years), multiparity (>4 prior pregnancies), and previous infertility treatment (which although important to document, do not significantly increase risk of adverse outcomes). Women were excluded from the study if they were at "genuinely high risk" (including multiple gestation). Those who were nominally "high risk" had significantly elevated levels of anxiety compared with women who were labelled "no risk," although the groups were clinically analogous. Simply being labelled "high risk" may provoke anxiety.

Regrettably, to date, no qualitative studies have investigated mothers' experiences of multiple pregnancy. The only quantitative study of psychological health in high-risk multiple pregnancy was a study by Maloni and colleagues in 2006, which investigated mothers on prescribed bed rest. As discussed below, bed rest on its own may be a source of psychological distress. The implications for maternal well-being of experiencing a high-risk multiple pregnancy alone (that is, without the additional stressor of prescribed bed rest) are unknown.

"MINOR DISCOMFORTS" OF MULTIPLE PREGNANCY FOR MOTHERS

As part of the Avon Longitudinal Study of Pregnancy and Childhood, Thorpe, Greenwood, and Goodenough surveyed 147 women pregnant with twins, and 11,061 pregnant with singletons. Study participants completed questionnaires, including health and emotional well-being items at twenty and thirty-two weeks' gestation. The authors found significantly poorer subjective physical health (particularly due to excessive vomiting), but not poorer emotional health among mothers pregnant with twins. Although the precise cause of pregnancy-related vomiting (morning sickness) remains unclear, it is speculated that placental hormones make a significant contribution. Even though the total placental mass in a twin gestation is slightly less than double that of a singleton placenta, it is nonetheless significantly greater (Pinar et al. 901); levels of pregnancy-associated hormones have been shown to be twice those of women pregnant with singletons at seventeen to nineteen weeks (Zheng et al. 555).

Pregnancy-related vomiting falling short of the threshold required for diagnosis of *hyperemesis gravidarum* (severe vomiting with weight loss) may nonetheless be highly distressing; a qualitative study of mothers of multiples with special needs included the words of one mother: "I'd been so sick with morning sickness, I thought nothing could've survived in there" (Bolch et al., "Multiple Birth Families" 507).

Other studies have corroborated the finding that mothers of multiples experience greater numbers of such "minor" discomforts during pregnancy than do mothers of singletons (Maloni, Margevicius, and Damato 115). These discomforts include symptoms such as indigestion and heartburn, back and hip pain, shortness of breath, and sleep disturbance. The effect of experiencing numerous unpleasant symptoms has been demonstrated to be multiplicative rather than additive (Lenz et al. 14). A brief appraisal of any online multiple pregnancy message board will confirm that although such common problems may be considered medically minor, their combined impact may indeed be profound. Even a straightforward multiple pregnancy may be physically and psychologically challenging.

MAJOR OBSTETRIC COMPLICATIONS

Campbell and Templeton reviewed the medical histories of 1,694 women pregnant with twin pregnancies and 71,851 with singletons between 1976 and 1999 in the Grampian region of Scotland. Mothers of twins were at significantly increased risk of severe vomiting, *anaemia* (insufficient numbers of red blood cells), premature detachment of the placenta from the wall of the uterus, *pre-eclampsia* (high blood pressure with protein in the urine), *eclampsia* (seizures related to high blood pressure), and blood clots. A woman enduring hyperemesis and anaemia, for example, experiences intractable vomiting, nausea, and fatigue. Such debilitation (which may begin early, and only end once the pregnancy ends) may have a lingering influence. Following the infants' birth, the focus shifts immediately from mother to babies, and in the anxiety of the first postnatal days and weeks, although understandably prioritizing her infants' health concerns, a mother may neglect her own need to recover from a considerable physical ordeal. Obstetric models of care do not generally include a period of rehabilitation for mothers of multiples.

PRESCRIBED BED REST

Mothers pregnant with multiples may be prescribed bed rest (often in hospital, with weight-bearing activities limited to walking to the toilet, if allowed at all) by their obstetric caregivers (Maloni, Margevicius, and Damato 115). Systematic reviews of the best available evidence (Cochrane Reviews) have found insufficient evidence to support or refute bed rest either in singleton (Sosa, Althabe, Belizan, and Bergel) or multiple pregnancies (Crowther and Han) as a means of preventing premature birth. Evidence is also lacking for benefits to twins in terms of neonatal morbidity or mortality (Ruiz, Brown, and Kirk 15). Nonetheless, the intervention continues to be widely recommended. Bigelow and Stone reported that up to 95 percent of obstetricians use antepartum activity restriction in some form (291). These authors argued that well-designed randomized controlled trials were necessary to conclusively determine the role of bed rest in specific obstetric populations. Although there may not be evidence for improved neonatal outcomes following prescribed bed rest, premature infants born *within* a tertiary level centre (as may occur if a mother is on inpatient bed rest) have significantly better outcomes than "outborn" infants (as would be the case if she were not) (Chien et al. 247), with immediate access to specialized care clearly implicated. In contrast, adverse physical and psychological consequences of bed rest for mothers are well documented. Physical deconditioning with loss of muscle mass and bone density, akin to that experienced by astronauts, occurs following a period of bed rest (Maloni 318). Maternal sleep duration and quality are diminished (Gallo and Lee 715).

Psychological complications of bed rest for mothers with multiple gestations have been both quantitatively (Maloni, Margevicius, and Damato) and qualitatively (Rubarth et al.) investigated. In these studies, antepartum "minor" physical and psychological symptoms were much more prevalent among multiple mothers after one week of bed rest than among mothers of singletons on bed rest (twenty-two symptoms experienced, compared with eight) (Maloni, Margevicius, and Damato 115).

In their discussion of psychological aspects of multiple pregnancy, Garel and colleagues stated: "When bed rest is ordered it is often taken badly and can bring on depression" ("Multiple Fetuses Pregnancy" 101). This assertion is supported by evidence. In 2006, Maloni and colleagues conducted a longitudinal repeated measures study involving thirty-one mothers of twins or triplets on antepartum bed rest. The authors found slightly higher levels of psychological distress compared with previous data from mothers of singletons, with 54.8 percent of the sample "at risk of depressive illness" at admission (scoring ≥ 16 on the Centre for Epidemiologic Studies Depression Scale [CES-D]) (Maloni, Margevicius, and

Damato 115). Levels of distress were highest at commencement of bed rest and diminished somewhat over time, commensurate with advancing gestational age and anticipated improved neonatal outcomes. Rubarth et al. conducted an ethnographic study of the experiences of eleven women on antepartum bed rest in the Midwestern United States, three of whom were pregnant with twins. Conclusions regarding bed rest in multiple pregnancy were not reported separately; however, two quotations from mothers of twins were cited: "We never really thought we would be at this point of just looking to simply 'survive.' We want healthy babies that we can take home with us right away," and "I know this time spent in the hospital is ultimately worth it. Giving our babies a better start to life—it's worth every tear, every moment of boredom, monotony, and sadness" (Rubarth et al. 402).

Our previous study of quality of life concerns among a group of 125 mothers of older multiples found that the experience of bed rest during pregnancy was significantly associated with elevated levels of maternal fatigue, on average more than five years after the event. Similarly, mothers who had given birth by Caesarean section were significantly more likely to report excessive fatigue than were women who had given birth vaginally (Bolch et al., "The MultiQOL Study" 418). Although far from conclusive, these findings do suggest that bed rest and surgical birth may have long term consequences for mothers of multiples.

BODY IMAGE AND MULTIPLE BIRTH

The term "body image" refers to an individual's conceptualization of her or his physical appearance, and is dependent on the interaction between thoughts, feelings, and perceived ideals within a social and cultural context (Australian Medical Association). The bodily changes associated with pregnancy sit starkly at odds with the prevailing "ideal" female form in occidental cultures (invariably slender; frequently childlike in appearance [Bordo 185]). Surveys have repeatedly demonstrated that most women of childbearing age are dissatisfied with their body and appearance. For many women, the physical changes of pregnancy, which are heightened by the presence of multiple fetuses, are genuinely alarming. On one online forum, a first-time prospective mother of twins lamented: "I'm 21 weeks with non ID twins and feel like a big fat whale!" ("Hardest Part About Having Twins").

A woman pregnant with twins has a similar appearance to a woman at term with a singleton pregnancy by the time she reaches her early third trimester (from twenty-eight weeks). At this point, she is likely to receive appraising comments from strangers such as "Any day now!" Although well-intentioned, such comments may add to her very real anxiety over possible premature birth. The babies could, indeed, arrive "any day now," but this would be ten weeks earlier than intended.

Optimal birthweight for twins (2500g) is associated with maternal weight gain of 18.2 to 20.5kg (40 to 45 lb.) (Luke 403). This is close to double the weight gain recommended for singleton pregnancies (11.5 to 16 kg or 25 to 35 lb.) (Rasmussen et al. 252). Such dramatic weight gain, combined with marked anatomical distortions required to accommodate multiple fetuses, leaves permanent marks on most women's postpartum bodies. The potential for negative postpartum body image to adversely affect maternal well-being has received relatively little academic attention (although body dissatisfaction at nine months has been found to be associated with poorer mental health in one study, which excluded mothers of multiples [Gjerdingen et al. 491]). Perceived loss of bodily integrity, due to changes associated with reproduction, may contribute to perinatal distress in some women. The potential for body dissatisfaction to adversely affect maternal mental health among mothers of multiples has not been specifically studied to date, although the possibility has been noted (e.g. "The future mother must accept the major deformation of her body. Some bear it proudly, but others find it difficult" [Garel, Charlemaine and Missonnier 101]).

Distress over physical changes imposed by multiple gestation may not be limited to the perinatal period either; mothers in our quality of life study who reported a diagnosis of a mental illness since their multiples' birth (on average, more than five years earlier) were significantly more likely to be distressed by physical changes resulting from their multiple pregnancy than were mothers who had not had a diagnosed mental health problem. This does not necessarily mean that physical changes *contributed to* their mental ill health (a depressed woman is more likely to judge her own body harshly); however, it is clear that some association exists. Physical consequences of multiple gestation are widely acknowledged in informal multiple birth peer support circles, where terms like "twin skin" (referring to loose and wrinkled abdominal skin), "twin tummy," and "apron" (referring to overhanging abdominal skin) are used. That some women are truly distressed by their altered appearance is clear from the following examples from different women: "My stomach is now sagging with extra skin / protruding / stretch marked and just horrible" ("Pregnant for the First Time"); "My stomach looks so bad.... Sometimes I am okay with it and sometimes it makes me want to cry" ("Hardest Part About Having Twins"); "It's been 10 months since I've had my twin babies, and I can honestly say my stomach has me very self-conscious and depressed" ("I Hate My Belly after Twins").

MULTIPLE CHILDBIRTH

Obstetric recommendations regarding the preferred mode of birth for multiples depend on many factors, including number of placentas and sacs, lie (position of the fetuses), gestation, estimated weights, caregiver skill and experience, and maternal preference. Likelihood of surgical birth (by Caesarean section) is increased for mothers of multiples. In Australia, two thirds of twins (and > 95 percent of triplets) are born by Caesarean section, compared with one third of singletons (Li et al. 33). Compared with vaginal birth, Caesarean birth is associated with significantly shorter maternal sleep duration and increased interruption to maternal sleep in the first postpartum week (Lee and Lee 109), and time to recovery may be prolonged (The Royal Australian and New Zealand College of Obstetricians and Gynaecologists 4).

Recently, a large randomized prospective trial of mode of delivery (Caesarean versus vaginal) involving 1,398 women and 2,795 fetuses with uncomplicated twin pregnancies, across 106 centres in 25 countries, demonstrated no significant difference in outcomes for twins born between 32 and 38+6 weeks (Barrett et al. 1295). Planned Caesarean section did not reduce risk of fetal or neonatal death or serious illness in straightforward twin births (first twin head down, close to term, and both fetuses known to be of a suitable size). This was somewhat contrary to expectations. Evidence is lacking regarding optimum management for more complicated twin births.

Surgical birth and use of obstetric interventions (including instrumental delivery—vacuum extraction or forceps) have been associated with increased risk of adverse psychological effects in new mothers (Fisher, Astbury, and Smith 728; Rowe-Murray and Fisher 1068), including post-traumatic stress disorder (Stramrood et al. 88). However, reported results are contradictory. A large observational study of 55,814 women in Norway found no association between mode of delivery and postnatal emotional disturbance at six months (Adams et al. 298). It is possible that the high-risk nature of a multiple pregnancy may render some women more comfortable accepting a surgical intervention that may offer their babies the best chance of a healthy outcome. This perspective is implied by online comments from women pregnant with multiples on the Australian Multiple Birth Association online forum: "As long as they come out nice and healthy, what does it matter?" ("Time for an Update").

None of the mothers in our previous qualitative study regretted having a Caesarean birth. They (and other mothers who gave birth vaginally) described being "struck, but not particularly troubled, by the sheer number of attendants at the birth, and frequently described their babies being 'whisked away'" (Bolch et al., "Multiple Birth Families" 507). The requirement for several sets of personnel and equipment is indeed peculiar to multiple birth.

For mothers of multiples giving birth vaginally, medical protocols are strictly adhered to (such as epidural anaesthesia, to allow for expedient manual removal of the second twin if necessary), which do not always provide for the psychological aspects of giving birth (Garel, Charlemaine, and Missonnier 99). Within subcultures in which maternal preferences surrounding birth are highly valued (as demonstrated by the popularity of the written "birth plan") such proscriptions can be experienced by some women as disempowering. As an example, one woman expecting twins asked an online multiples support group for samples of twin birth plans, and was met with the following response: "My doc just laughs at birth plans. He says you can't plan a twin birth, there are just too many variables" ("Subconscious Favouritism").

BECOMING A MOTHER FOR THE FIRST TIME WHILE BECOMING A MOTHER OF MULTIPLES

In a large study commissioned by TAMBA (the Twins and Multiple Births Association—the United Kingdom's multiple birth peer support group), data from the Family Resources Survey were analysed (McKay). This study compared demographic and other characteristics of 581 families with twins, 14 with triplets, and 25,000 without multiple birth children, born in 2000 and 2001. Nearly half of all the mothers of multiples are making the transition to parenthood at the same time as they are becoming parents of multiple birth children (that is, multiples are their first children).

Becoming a mother requires psychological and social adjustments, many of which are experienced as losses (Barclay and Lloyd), including the loss of autonomy and discretionary time and the time to maintain other relationships as well as the loss of income, control, personal liberty, sense of self, confidence, and self-esteem (Barclay et al. 722). Given existing evidence of psychosocial stress associated with the transition to motherhood in general, it is likely that first-time mothers of multiples experience greater adjustment challenges than those who already have children. Among a group of 103 mothers of twins, first-time mothers were shown to have significantly greater stress related to parenting competence, health, and partner relationships than did mothers of twins who had older children (Colpin and Vandemeulebroecke 3133). Use of assisted conception was associated with increased levels of stress for first-time mothers.

A study conducted in Israel between 2003 and 2004 shed further light on maternal adaptation to multiple birth. Findler and colleagues collected demographic and psychosocial data at birth and at twelve months post-birth from seventy mothers of premature twins, and seventy-eight mothers of twins born at term. First-time mothers of twins born at term enjoyed superior mental health outcomes to both mothers of twins born prematurely, and mothers with previous children. The authors concluded:

16

> First time mothers of full-term twins enjoy a more facilitating
> environment which allows them to dedicate themselves
> fully to the new challenge, without being torn between the
> demands of the newborns and those of other children on
> the one hand, and without suffering the uncertainty and
> anxieties related to the potential risks of premature infants
> on the other. (Findler, Taubman-Ben-Ari, and Jacob 53)

In the multiple birth peer support context, it is recognized that
lack of experience has both advantages and disadvantages. While
a first-time mother may not have the practical knowledge that
comes from experience, her only frame of reference is having two
(or more) infants simultaneously: "You don't know any different,
you just see 2 as normal and you get very efficient very quickly.
You learn to be organised. This is normal for me because I don't
know what a singleton feels like" ("Did Anyone").

In our study of quality of life of mothers of multiples, we found no
difference between quality of life of first-time mothers of multiples
and those who already had children (Bolch et al., "The MultiQOL
Study" 418). We did however identify several differences in mothers'
perception of the meaning of their multiples' birth and in some
of their attitudes regarding their children. First-time mothers of
multiples were more likely to agree that having multiples had
given them an "instant family" (particularly when their children
were of different sexes). They enjoyed having a more "hands on"
parenting role than they had anticipated but mourned the loss of
their imagined relationship with a "single" child (this was true
even for those who went on to have a singleton). Mothers with
a previous singleton felt social restrictions imposed by having
multiples more keenly than did first-time mothers and were more
troubled by the household chaos generated by their multiple birth
children.

NEONATAL INTENSIVE CARE AND SPECIAL CARE OF MULTIPLES

Adaptation to mothering may be complicated by the experience of
giving birth prematurely to a medically fragile infant. The majority
of twins (57.3 percent in the authors' home country, Australia),

17

and all higher order multiples, are born prematurely (prior to thirty-seven weeks) (Li et al. 33), compared with 6.7 percent of singletons. Multiples are particularly heavily overrepresented at very early gestations (before thirty-two weeks) when infants' requirements for medical intervention and support are greater and a favourable outcome is much less certain. Premature and sick newborns look startlingly different to healthy term newborns. Several mothers in our qualitative study described feeling horrified by their babies' initial appearance: "You look TERRIBLE! And ugly! And where's my big, fat, beautiful babies?" (Bolch et al., "Multiple Birth Families" 508).

Our study also found that for some mothers of multiples, the contrast between their postnatal experience (involving immediate removal and transfer of their babies to intensive care) and that of term, singleton mothers (immediate contact with their baby, who then roomed in) could be particularly distressing. In one mother's words, "The first night was really quite revolting, being in this room with five other women who all had their babies with them, and sitting there going 'Where are MY babies?' And hating that feeling" (Bolch et al., "Multiple Birth Families" 507).

In a qualitative study of mothering in two Australian Special Care Nurseries (SCNs) involving interviews with twenty-eight mothers and twenty nursery staff, Fenwick, Barclay and Schmied described the work done by mothers in getting to know their premature and/ or ill infants and learning the rules of life in the nursery. Mothers engaged in activities aimed at achieving intimate knowledge of their infant and attempted to apply the information in establishing and consolidating their role of "mother," while under the supervision of the nursery staff. Our research suggests that the experience of mothers of multiples is similar, with additional complications imposed by the twin relationship (such as physical separation of infants from each other within the nursery, forcing mothers to choose one child over another): "They were in different sections. So we had to choose who to visit first. That still upsets me. How was I meant to choose?" (Bolch et al., "Multiple Birth Families" 512).

Social support—an interpersonal transaction involving both emotional and instrumental (tangible) assistance (Wandersman, Wandersman, and Kahn)—has been identified as an important element of maternal well-being following premature birth. Singer et al. (521) conducted a longitudinal study of risk factors and stress and coping among mothers of term-born versus very low birth weight (VLBW) infants. For the VLBW group, the impacts of financial and general parenting stress were buffered by practical and emotional support from friends, family, and a partner.

Eiser et al. in the United Kingdom compared measures of mother and child quality of life, from 126 term and 91 premature infants, during the child's second year. Both maternal and child quality of life were more likely to be poor in the premature group in the child's second year, compared with term-born children and their mothers. One possible explanation suggested by the authors was that mothers of prematurely born infants are more likely to perceive their children as vulnerable and may adjust their parenting accordingly, being cautious about new experiences and therefore having reduced enjoyment of life.

A study by Allen et al., which took medical fragility into account, concluded that higher perceived vulnerability was associated with greater health care use and with maternal anxiety at discharge. Distinction is seldom drawn between a mother who *inappropriately* perceives her child as vulnerable (for example, following simple phototherapy for jaundice) compared with the anxiety experienced by the mother of a survivor of extreme prematurity, who is left with chronic lung disease, and regarding whom doctors have advised minimal social contact to prevent respiratory infections. In both situations, the family is described as suffering from "vulnerable child syndrome" (American Thoracic Society)—a somewhat problematic term, which may be perceived as disparaging by families to whom it is applied. "Vulnerable child syndrome" has been identified in 17 percent of non-urgent presentations to emergency departments (Chambers, Mahabee-Gittens, and Leonard 1009). In this study, the presence of "vulnerable child syndrome" was associated with previous complicated pregnancy or delivery, prematurity, poor child and maternal mental health, and child development problems. Although the question has not been explored, it is likely that the "vulnerable child" dynamic influences the early post-hospital days of many multiple birth families; we found evidence of intense, almost phobic, fear of infection following time in neonatal intensive care

19

and difficulty relinquishing care to others (Bolch et al., "Multiple Birth Families" 508).

Despite the prevalence of multiple birth among premature infants, the experiences of mothers of multiple birth infants in neonatal intensive care have not yet been studied specifically. Mothers of multiples are more likely to have experienced risk factors associated with "vulnerable child syndrome" (complicated pregnancy or delivery, prematurity, poor child and maternal mental health, and child development problems). It is likely that "vulnerable child(ren) syndrome" is a factor in postnatal anxiety among some mothers of premature multiples; however, this has not been documented. The practical and emotional difficulties for mothers tending to multiple infants in Neonatal Intensive or Special Care have been acknowledged in parenting support publications (Gromada and Hurlburt; Bowman and Ryan).

STAGGERED DISCHARGE FROM HOSPITAL

Specific to the multiple birth circumstance is "staggered discharge," in which one (or more) multiple birth infants is discharged from hospital days, weeks, or even months before her or his co-multiple/s. For a new mother of twins, this means that she will be providing care to a newborn (often prematurely-born) infant who is at home, while she travels to and from hospital to visit and care for a co-multiple. If her hospitalized infant is receiving breastmilk, she will also be expressing and transporting her milk. Research conducted during the 1970s and 1980s suggested that parents were likely to form a preference for the infant discharged from hospital first and that such parental preference was maintained through to adolescence (Hay, "Adolescent Twins and Secondary Schooling" 119). These studies were, however, with small samples and are not representative of twins in general (involving only 27 pairs of female monozygotic twins). The validity of extrapolating from these studies to how parents of twins may regard their children today is debatable. In the past, parents of twins were often advised to take one twin home while leaving the other in hospital to become accustomed to infant care (Hay and O'Brien 242). Today's parents are highly unlikely to be offered the opportunity to take one twin home, simply for "practice," but intense pressure on resources, with fewer neonatal beds being available in nurseries than are needed, means a medically stable twin is nonetheless likely to be discharged before his or her less stable co-twin. There are no current data on parents' experience of staggered discharge of multiples and no studies at all regarding staggered discharge of male monozygotic, or any dizygotic twins.

IMPLICATIONS OF ATYPICAL ANTENATAL COURSE AND BIRTH FOR POSTNATAL MOTHERS

Sleep Disturbance, Fatigue, and Mothers of Multiples

New mothers (of singletons) are frequently advised to "rest when the baby rests" during the day to minimize fatigue. Mothers of twins may be unable to follow this advice, given the presence of another wakeful baby needing care. Night time awakenings may be doubled (or tripled) and multiples sharing a room may wake each other. Elevated fatigue among mothers of twins is not just due to poor sleep; during waking hours, caregiving requirements are multiplied, diminishing time that might otherwise be spent resting or playing and interacting with the babies.

In 2008, Damato and Burant demonstrated significant sleep disturbance among eight sets of first-time parents of twins over the first twenty postnatal weeks. Both fewer hours of sleep and increased nocturnal awakenings, compared with singleton parents, were found. Although results from such a small sample are not generalizable, some important information was obtained. Reported levels of fatigue failed to decline over the study period, despite increases in nocturnal sleep, and fewer night awakenings. In a 2010 study, McKay found that 64 percent of mothers of nine-month-old twins felt tired most or all of the time, compared with 49 percent of mothers of singletons (7). In a Taiwanese study, in which 296 mothers of twins were interviewed regarding perceived problems associated with raising twins, the most frequently volunteered difficulty (49 percent) was inadequate maternal sleep (Chang 501).

Research into the mental health of mothers of multiples has not explicitly considered the association between chronic sleep deprivation and depressive symptoms. Disturbed sleep is a symptom of both depression (with early morning waking being typical) and anxiety (with delayed sleep onset). However, sleep deprivation is also causally implicated in mental health problems. The relationships among depression, anxiety, and fatigue in the perinatal period are complex and poorly understood, but the phenomena are highly correlated (Swanson et al. 553).

Chronic sleep deprivation has been shown to induce structural changes to the brain, particularly to the hippocampus, in animal models (Novati et al. 145). These changes result in physiological and neurobiological changes, which are very similar to those seen in people who are depressed. Chronic fragmentation of sleep (intermittent interruption) has been shown to induce equally significant changes (Guzman-Marin et al. 325). It is likely that sleep deprivation has a "sensitizing" effect that *contributes* to the development of mood disorders, rather than simply being a symptom of them (Meerlo et al. 187). A review of studies of primary insomnia (that is, insomnia *not* associated with another physical or mental condition) found an unambiguous association between insomnia and subsequent increased risk of depression (Riemann and Voderholzer 255).

Fatigue in new parents is a considerable problem but its contribution to perinatal mental ill health has been inadequately explored to date (Ross, Murray, and Steiner). Fatigue differs from normal tiredness (relieved by adequate rest), in that it is "more severe, enduring and persistent" (Giallo et al. 69). The association between unsettled infant behaviour, maternal fatigue, and new onset of maternal depressive symptoms was documented by Dennis and Ross (187). They studied mothers who did *not* have depressive symptoms one week postpartum, and identified associations among those who subsequently became depressed at four and eight weeks. Depressed mothers were significantly more likely than those who were not depressed to report that their baby cried often, did not sleep well, and woke them three times or more between 10:00 p.m. and 6:00 a.m., and that they had received fewer than six hours of sleep on at least one day in the past week. Although this is not conclusive proof that caring for a crying, wakeful baby contributes to depression, these mothers were not depressed *until* they were exposed to this experience.

Several studies have offered evidence that fatigue and depression are distinct but related concepts (Giallo et al.; Fisher, Feekery, and Rowe-Murray). One study of mothers of children seeking treatment for sleep problems found that 40 percent of mothers reported depressive symptoms in the clinical range. Following resolution of their child's sleeping problems, only 4.3 percent scored in the "depressed" range. The authors concluded that a significant proportion of women are misdiagnosed with depression, when they are suffering from chronic sleep deprivation (Armstrong et al. 260). This study demonstrated that fatigue is strongly implicated in depressive symptoms among mothers of infants attending unsettled baby clinics. It is highly likely that fatigue is a significant contributor to the elevated rates of depression identified among mothers of multiples.

CHALLENGES OF THE NEWBORN PERIOD AND INFANCY: PRACTICAL CARE NEEDS

Investigators have found that mothers of multiples appear to have less enjoyment in their babies than mothers of singletons (Holditch-Davis, Roberts, and Sandelowski). This conclusion might not be surprising given the results of one survey that reported that caregiving takes twenty-eight hours and twelve minutes per day ("Having Twins and Triplets") and, for all multiples, involves multiple feeds and nappy changes (Gromada and Hurlburt 65). Although total feeds per day decline with time—from nineteen at two weeks post-discharge of twins from hospital to thirteen at twenty weeks (Damato and Burant 742)—at all ages, basic care needs are increased. Until mother and babies learn to tandem (simultaneously) feed, feeds are often given separately. Many mothers express breastmilk mechanically to increase or maintain supply (up to three hours per day if guidelines are followed) (Gromada and Hurlburt 66).

Once multiple infants become mobile, they explore independently, and supervision becomes paramount. Investigating caregiving implications of fatigue among mothers with debilitating chronic illnesses (rheumatoid arthritis and multiple sclerosis), White and colleagues found that fatigue reduced maternal monitoring of children (325). Multiple birth children experience increased levels of hospitalization for accidental injuries (Roudsari et al. 121), perhaps attributable in part to maternal fatigue. Investigating early parenting behaviours of mothers of twins, Robin and colleagues found that non-fatigued mothers (who were more likely to receive outside help) were more able to individualize the care of their multiples and to be flexible than were chronically depressed and fatigued mothers ("Childcare Patterns" 453).

MOTHERING OUTSIDE THE NORM

In well-resourced high-income countries, the informal multi-generational networks of women that, historically, imparted advice regarding mothering and provided opportunities to learn by observation have eroded. Many governments have now introduced early parenting education classes, facilitated by a nurse educator. For example, in Victoria, Australia, first-time mothers are allocated to a "new mothers group," which is coordinated by local government services. Mothers and their infants meet weekly for six weeks at a local centre to receive infant care education, delivered by a trained maternal and child health nurse.

First-time mothers of multiples are usually allocated to a group on the basis of their babies' actual date of birth, which (if born prematurely) may be weeks earlier than their expected date. This means that, should she manage to attend the group, her babies will appear significantly delayed compared with term, singleton babies. It is unusual for more than one mother of multiples to be in a group. Anecdotes from members of online parenting forums are consistent:

> I didn't even make it to the third session at the centre as the second door was always bolted locked and they made me feel like such a hassle for having to unlock it and open the door for me to get a double pram in. And the looks I would get from the other mothers (ones of horror or distaste) really made me uncomfortable. ("Parents Group")

> I felt like I had NOTHING in common with anyone else.

They talked about how hard the first few months have been, how they had no time to themselves, how demanding their babies were ... All true I'm sure, but I just couldn't help sitting there thinking "Oh my God, none of you have the faintest idea what hard is, stop complaining!" I also spent the whole time feeding, settling etc. while they were enjoying coffee. ("Mothers Group, Is It Worth It?")

SOCIAL STIGMA, BOUNDARY TRANSGRESSIONS, AND INTRUSIVE QUESTIONING

Social and cultural contexts are relevant because parenting does not occur in a vacuum. For most parents of multiples, twin or triplet parenthood comes unexpectedly, and prior to conception, they might have shared common misapprehensions about the desirability and unusual nature of multiples. Sociologist Erving Goffman defined "social stigma" as "the process by which the reaction of others spoils normal identity" (qtd. in Nettleton 95). Mothers of multiples are at increased risk of experiencing social stigma (Ellison and Hall; Roca-de Bes, Gutierrez-Maldonado, and Gris-Martínez), particularly because of the widespread assumption that multiple gestation is inevitably the result of conception with assisted reproductive technologies (ART), especially in vitro fertilization. Although ART-associated multiple births were prevalent in the recent past, they never represented the majority of *twin* births, even in North America (where in 2011, 36 percent of twins resulted from ART [Kulkarni et al.]). North America has been slow to adopt recommended changes to reproductive technology practice that were instituted in Australia and the United Kingdom in the mid-2000s (in particular transfer of one rather than multiple embryos) and led to a decline in multiple birth in those countries. Currently in Australia, fewer than 20 percent of multiples are conceived with medical assistance (Umstad et al. 158). Triplets and other higher order multiples are more likely to be conceived with assistance than are twins; even so, in Australia, fewer than 20 percent follow IVF whereas in North America, it is 77 percent.

Mothers of multiple birth infants are subjected to public scrutiny and intrusive questioning to a degree that surprises most and offends many. These can be experienced as boundary violations, in which the mother's right to privacy is transgressed. One woman described being stopped by strangers eighteen times during a fifty minute shopping trip ("Things Not to Say to a Twin Mum"). Strangers may ask if her children are "natural" (that is, conceived spontaneously) or with medical assistance. Raj and Morley explored the attitudes of Australian parents of multiples to sharing information regarding their children's conception, particularly with medical researchers. One participant offered: "When pregnant I was amazed at people in the street asking me if they were IVF—I responded with 'Are you asking me if we had sex to conceive?' Essentially they are asking me about my sex life. It is invasive, rude, and irrelevant" (888).

Some mothers of multiples respond to the question "Were they IVF?" more assertively, for example: "No, they were S.E.X." ("IVF or Natural"). Even the seemingly innocuous question "Do twins run in your family?" asks indirectly about conception. Ellison and Hall documented widespread experiences of social stigma among parents of ART-conceived multiples (405) and Raj and Morley demonstrated that stigma extends to all parents of multiples, regardless of mode of conception (886).

This experience parallels that of mothers in same-sex relationships, who are questioned similarly about intimate information by strangers:

> Twin parents should hang out with same sex parents more often. This level of intrusive questioning is seen as perfectly acceptable towards my wife and I [sic]. Except people want to know who is the "real" mother. My answer is "we both are." Or they want to know if the kids look like their father, because they're fishing for information about my family that is none of their business. ("Twin Mums are Freaks of Nature")

Complex and personal family planning decisions may be glibly summarized:

> We get stopped quite a lot, as you do with twins, and get comments about "how lucky" we are to have a "pigeon

pair" because "now you're finished". And that bugs me too. Because I don't like people assuming that just because we have a girl and a boy, that necessarily completes things for me. ("Pigeon Pair")

Frequently, mothers of multiples are told that "*My* two were born (X) months apart—that's just as hard as (or harder than) having twins" (Fierro, "Is Having Twins the Same"). Comments and observations might be kindly meant and intended as humorous such as the following: "Better you than me!" (Holditch-Davis, Roberts, and Sandelowski 206); "I don't know how you do it!"—as though mothers have a choice; or the ubiquitous "You've got your hands full!" ("Things Not to Say to a Twin Mum"). However, when offered to a tired mother with two screaming toddlers at a supermarket checkout, such comments are usually experienced as unempathic and critical. Many mothers of boy-girl twins are asked to explain precisely *why* their children aren't identical. The term "double trouble" becomes potentially harmful rather than merely irritating when the children are old enough to understand its meaning. "Which one's your favourite?" is surpassed only by "So which one's the evil twin?" for insensitivity ("Things Not to Say to a Twin Mum").

Metaphorical boundary transgression (such as unwelcome questioning) is frequently accompanied by *physical* boundary transgression, in which strangers enter the personal space of the multiple infants and touch them. Although this occurs with singleton infants, the novelty of multiples seems to encourage this behaviour. "I also didn't like the way complete strangers felt some sort of entitlement to come over ... they get right down into the babies' faces, touch them and look truly insulted and 'hmpff' me when I say 'excuse me, please don't touch my children'" ("Which One Is the Aggressive One?"). While these encounters may appear humorous, repeated exposure contributes to self-perceptions of being outside the "norm."

THE ROLE OF MULTIPLE BIRTH PEER SUPPORT GROUPS

A sense of affiliation or belonging to a group with others is considered a basic human need (Maslow). Social researchers have observed that people tend to seek group affiliation under circumstances of actual or anticipated stress (Wandersman, Wandersman, and Kahn 333). The only place mothers of multiples may feel that they belong is among others with similar lived experiences. This reality is exemplified by the mottos of several organizations: Irish Multiple Birth Association (IMBA): "parents helping parents"; Multiples of America: "connecting and supporting multiple birth families"; or Australian Multiple Birth Association (AMBA): "support from those who know." As membership of peer support groups is voluntary, they represent a self-selected subset of parents of multiples, and it is unclear whether they are representative of parents of multiples in general. We found that mothers of multiples with additional needs, who diverged from the "healthy term multiples" narrative, were less likely to find group membership helpful. As one mother of twins born at twenty-four weeks said, "Their twins were all born at thirty-seven weeks, you know. So we found we actually felt really out of place, and we've never been back". Another mother of twins with cerebral palsy related "I did go [to the multiple birth group]. There was just no one there with disabilities, it just put me off" (Bolch et al., "Multiple Birth Families" 511).

UNEQUAL OPPORTUNITIES

There have been sustained arguments for additional parenting education and practical support for multiple birth families, particularly in the early months (Neifert and Thorpe; Leonard; Nys et al.; Bryan, "The Impact of Multiple Preterm Births on the Family"; McKay). Mothers of multiple birth children rarely have access to early parenting education or assistance that is specific to their needs. Experiences of discrimination (unfavourable treatment because of a personal characteristic) and marginalization are detrimental to mental health (Kessler, Mickelson, and Williams 208). Discrimination on the basis of parental or carer status or family responsibilities is unlawful in many jurisdictions (e.g., state laws covering "Family Responsibilities Discrimination" in parts of U.S. [Workplace Fairness]; the 1984 *Sex Discrimination Act* [Australian Human Rights Commission]).

Many public amenities (including public transport, medical premises, and shops) are not designed for physical access of a double pram (which is, by necessity, wider than a standard pram and is also wider than a wheelchair). Mothers are unable to take twins to group activities that require one carer per child, which increases social isolation, as explained by one mother on an online forum: "I called a local gymnastics school that offers a kiddie gym class. I told her I had twins and she basically told me not to try—it wouldn't work" ("Gymboree—Not Possible with 18mo Twins?").

ECONOMIC AND EMPLOYMENT IMPLICATIONS
OF MULTIPLE BIRTH

The financial costs of a multiple birth to the family are considerable. Some achieve pregnancy following costly infertility treatment (Fisher and Stocky 506), but regardless of mode of conception, there are needs for larger car(s), housing, furniture, clothing, nappies, and, frequently, formula (McKay 6), with costs that are incurred over a short time. Parents cannot re-use equipment or clothing as they might with children born consecutively, and total costs of raising multiples are higher.

Despite this, and contrary to a popular misconception, there is generally no entitlement for financial support on the grounds of multiple birth ("Practical Help and Financial Factsheet"). Even if available, parents of twins can be excluded. In the Australian social protection system, for example, there is a modest "multiple birth allowance," that was granted to parents of triplets but not twins in 2007.

In 2010, TAMBA (McKay) commissioned an investigation of the direct and indirect costs to families of having multiples. They experience significantly greater financial stress and material deprivation (poverty), have to spend more of their savings, and are worse off financially compared to the year preceding the birth than parents of singletons (8). Fathers of multiples more often work overtime to meet increased household financial needs, yet they have to also contribute more to caregiving and household work. Mothers of multiples in McKay's study took longer than mothers of singletons to return to paid employment (9). Centre-based child

29

care for twins is less accessible and more likely to be provided by a partner or paid nanny and costs are doubled.

Paid and unpaid maternity leave protect women's mental health (Chatterji and Markowitz 61), but the psychological benefits and hazards of maternal paid employment are complex to discern. Paid employment improves access to financial resources and collegial interactions and can enhance personal competence, but poor working conditions may jeopardize well-being (Cooklin et al. 222) and exacerbate conflict within the family. The costs of "outsourced" care for two or more children can render paid work uneconomic. Another mother of twins described her circumstances:

> I'm a stay at home mother, and I love the time I get to spend with my girls, but I would also like to have a part time job to allow me to see other people and have an identity outside of being mother and wife. But unless child care costs come down, then I just can't afford to go to work. ("Did Anyone")

In Israel, Baor and Soskolne found that mothers of IVF-conceived twins who were in paid employment experienced lower levels of stress than those who were unemployed; the authors speculated that employment may be a "coping resource" for such mothers (260). Resuming paid work presents particular dilemmas when health care benefits are tied to employment, for example in North America.

SELF-EFFICACY, SOCIAL SUPPORT, AND MATERNAL SENSE OF COMPETENCE

Maternal self-efficacy refers to a mother's belief in her ability to effectively manage the tasks and situations of motherhood (Gross and Rocissano 19). Both practical and emotional support may enhance maternal self-efficacy by providing opportunities and resources so that the mother can meet her infant's needs more easily, and recognize and value her own efforts. In a study of 410 first-time mothers of singletons at six weeks postpartum, poor maternal self-efficacy and perceived low levels of social support predicted postnatal depression (Leahy-Warren, McCarthy, and Corcoran 388).

McKay reported that mothers of infant twins were significantly less likely to feel "very competent and confident" looking after their children than were mothers of singletons (7). Persistent infant crying has been associated with diminished maternal sense of competence (Megel et al. 144). A mother of multiples is limited in her ability to respond immediately to two or more crying infants. It is unsurprising that maternal competence is undermined, which can cause considerable distress: "The hardest part is the guilt I feel when I know they both need to be held and I can only hold one" ("Hardest part about having twins").

Today's mothers of multiples are further compromised by the influential contemporary paradigm that holds that allowing an infant to cry *at all* is damaging: "We know now that leaving babies to cry is a good way to make a less intelligent, less healthy but more anxious, uncooperative and alienated person who can pass the same or worse traits on to the next generation" (Narvaez).

The tasks of establishing a maternal identity and developing confidence in the maternal role may be additionally complicated by premature birth (Lupton and Fenwick; Black, Holditch-Davis, and Miles). In the neonatal intensive care and special care settings, infants appear fragile and a mother's every action is open to the scrutiny of professionals. The challenge of establishing maternal identity and sense of competence in the context of premature *multiple* birth is greater still.

ATTACHMENT THEORY, BONDING, AND MULTIPLE BIRTH

The central premise of Bowlby and Ainsworth's attachment theory, describing the parent-infant relationship, was concisely summarized by Eells: "Affectional bonds between individuals and patterns of early life interactions between caregivers and children produce internal working models that serve as templates guiding interpersonal expectations and behaviors in later relationships" (132).

In general, "caregivers" are presumed to be "mothers." The quality of a child's attachment is believed to depend primarily on the mother's ability to respond sensitively to the child's signals (the "sensitivity hypothesis") (Ainsworth, Blehar, Waters, and Wall). Secure attachment in infancy is believed to predict adults who are more socially and emotionally competent than insecurely attached infants (the "competence hypothesis"). Infants who feel sufficiently protected and comforted by their mother's presence are believed to be more likely to explore their environments (the "secure base hypothesis") (Rothbaum et al. 1095). Failure of attachment between mother and infant in the first two years is hypothesized to lead to serious and irreversible consequences, including "affectionless psychopathy" (inability to show affection or concern for others), according to the "maternal deprivation" hypothesis (McLeod).

Critics, including Billings (207), argue that such theories are burdensome to women, "mother blaming," or biased towards studying mothers', but not fathers', contributions to child and adolescent maladjustment, and do not consider the gendered context in which birth and early parenting occur (Phares 656). Rothbaum and colleagues also criticize Western sociocultural biases. In a comparison of North American and Japanese parenting styles, they observed: "When U.S. parents care for their babies in ways valued by Japanese parents, they are considered insensitive, and their babies are found to be insecurely attached" (1097). Japanese caregiving practices to keep their children close, anticipate their needs, minimize stressors, and promote dependency can be considered "maladaptive" in comparison with the open communication style and individuality of the "secure" Western child. The authors conclude that "Attachment theory is infused with cultural assumptions, leading to misguided interpretation of research findings and unfortunate consequences for assessment, intervention, and intercultural understanding" (Rothbaum et al. 1102).

The application of attachment theory, which emerges from the psychoanalytic tradition, to the multiple birth situation (which, in many salient ways, *is* a different culture) is potentially problematic. Attachment in this context has been conceptualized as "triadic" (Robin, Josse, and Tourrette 151): a mother forms an attachment to each of her twins separately and to the twins as a "unit." Barton and Strosberg observed triadic conversational interactions between four mothers and their two-year-old twins, but applying this to relationships is contentious. Robin et al. (151) observed that 15 percent of mothers of two-month-old twins synchronized their feeding schedules and interpreted this as indicating that mothers' regarded their twins as a unit. In 1968, Bowlby proposed that attachment was "monotropic" and that "attachment can only take place for one infant at a time" (Robin et al., "Mother-Twin Interaction During Early Childhood" 1). It has been stated that, optimally, "parents attach to one infant only" (Thomas 233).

This paradigm, which lacks a strong evidence base, has remained largely unchallenged. It is inconsistent with discourse within the multiple birth community, in which transient and shifting preferences are acknowledged as commonplace and tend to be based on which child is least challenging at the time. For example, "You won't *love* one more, but you may *like* one more than the other at times, based on who the easier baby is"; or "I don't have a favorite, but whoever is not crying is my favorite in that moment" ("Subconscious Favouritism"). The concept of monotropic attachment is also inconsistent with the small amount of qualitative information, from mothers of multiples, who have reported an ability to form attachments to more than one infant simultaneously (Abbink et al. 411). Holditch-Davis et al. found that "All mothers and most fathers reported that they possessed equal feelings for both (or all) of the infants" (208). Cook et al found "no significant differences between groups (twins versus singletons) in maternal warmth or emotional involvement" (3245).

Characterizations of mothers of multiples in the attachment literature have tended to be harsh. Robin and colleagues reported their interpretations of interviews with fourteen mothers of triplets within a year of birth:

This initial shock [of diagnosis] is replaced by a pregnancy which tends to be devolved to a level of hypochondriac complaints concerning their bodies.... In multiple pregnancies there is a striking lack of the heightened inward sensitivity that occurs during singleton pregnancies

> ... The shock of reality is so intense that mothers of triplets
> become totally insensitive to [their infants'] emotional
> distress. ("Maternal Adjustment to a Multiple Birth" 3-8)

Robin and colleagues draw a parallel between some maternal preferences for one child, and their previous inability to perceive all multiples moving in utero ("Maternal Adjustment to a Multiple Birth" 9). Elsewhere, the responsibility of the mother for her multiples' psychological health is made explicit: "It is very much up to the mother to ensure that the constant presence of a third individual is not experienced as parasitism by the other twin" (Athanassiou 329). Mothers of multiples who have access to practical help also risk damaging their children: "When there is an increase in the number of carers, the secure base may be less secure" (Sandbank 162). Mothers of multiples reading these assertions could be forgiven for feeling somewhat dispirited.

Attachment styles in this situation have been described as "preferential" (with the parent—generally the mother—preferring one infant over the other/s), alternating (switching preference between children), or "unit bonding" (in which children are managed and it has been presumed, conceptualized by the parent as a "unit") (Gromada and Hurlburt 86-89). A further criticism of much "attachment" literature about mothers and twins is that it has been prone to two errors: first, inferring maternal preference from observed behaviours (such as picking up or patting); and second, comparing the care given to multiples with that for singletons, using a "per child" calculation rather than summing interactions with all infants.

The potential for misattribution of maternal feelings from actions is amplified because of the increased practical care requirements. A woman who adapts to feeding her twins by propping their bottles rather than cradling them may be revealing more about the need for efficient task completion than her "attachment" to either child. Rothbaum and colleagues argue in their critique of attachment theory that "Relationships in other cultures are not inferior but instead are adaptations to different circumstances" (1101).

It appears overall that explorations of mothering multiples have been governed by a singleton norm that positions the mothers as performing an inferior version of "normal" mothering. Attachment theorists are yet to consider that multiple birth mothers and children may find different but nonetheless healthy ways of accommodating unusual circumstances.

THE MEDICAL MODEL OF POSTNATAL DEPRESSION
AND THE PROBLEM OF DEFINITION

Postnatal psychological distress is commonly conceptualized within a medical model, which considers it a mental illness (Barclay and Lloyd 136). It is presumed to result from abnormal levels of neurotransmitters, particularly serotonin, which can influence mood (Noble 49), and that post-birth hormonal changes are the causal link (Studd and Nappi 42). Postnatal depression (PND) is considered distinct from the early emotional lability that can follow birth, the "baby blues," which up to 80 percent of women (in Western populations) experience. PND also differs from the rare, but serious postnatal psychosis, which follows 0.1% to 0.2% of births (Hübner-Liebermann, Hausner, and Wittmann 420). Postnatal psychosis develops rapidly, within four weeks of birth, and is characterized by disturbances of thinking and behaviour and is conceptualized as an episode of bipolar disorder (Sit, Rothschild, and Wisner 352).

Under the medical model, individuals are categorized on the basis of diagnostic criteria as being "well" or "unwell." However, not all distress following childbirth meets criteria for major depression descriptive criteria for postnatal depression.

SYMPTOMS OF POSTNATAL DEPRESSION

Although the condition is commonly studied, diagnosed, and managed, the case for "postnatal depression" as a conceptually distinct entity, which is clearly distinguishable from generic "depression," is unclear. The *Diagnostic and Statistical Manual of Mental Disorders* (fifth edition) does not define postnatal depression as a distinct entity but considers it a variant of major depression (American Psychiatric Association 150). DSM-5 criteria for a diagnosis of postnatal depression are the same as those for major depressive episode, with the temporal qualifier of "onset within 4 weeks of delivery." In general use, and in much of the clinical research, the definition of postnatal depression is broadened to include major depression with onset within twelve months of birth (Gjerdingen and Yawn 280). Symptoms include depressed mood and markedly diminished pleasure in activities for at least two weeks and at least four of the following: significant weight loss or gain or change in appetite; sleep disturbance; objective psychomotor agitation or slowing; fatigue; feelings of worthlessness or excessive guilt; poor concentration or difficulty making decisions; and suicidal thoughts (American Psychiatric Association).

Changes associated with new motherhood (such as weight loss and sleep disturbance) complicate application of these criteria. In the postnatal context, experts have suggested that sleep disturbance should be regarded as a symptom only if it is unrelated to the infant's needs—a woman may additionally fear being alone, she may be irritable and feel unable to cope, and may fear harming the baby (Post and Antenatal Depression Association, 2012). Further features such as ambivalence towards the child, fear of failure or feelings of inadequacy as a mother have also been proposed (Hübner-Liebermann, Hausner, and Wittmann 420).

RISK FACTORS FOR POSTNATAL DEPRESSION

One of the strongest predictors of postnatal depression is a personal history of depression, and risk of depression correlates with severity of previous episodes (Topiwala, Hothi, and Ebmeier 15). The variables demonstrated in a large systematic review to be significantly associated with antenatal and postnatal depression in mothers are listed in Table One.

A recent systematic review of evidence regarding risk factors for postnatal depression among mothers of premature and low-birthweight infants identified that sustained depression was associated with greater degree of prematurity, lower birthweight, ongoing concerns about the health and development of the infant, and perceived lack of social support (Vigod et al. 540). Multiple birth increases risk of each of these parameters.

MOTHERS OF MULTIPLES AND DEPRESSION

Elevated levels of depression among mothers of multiples are well recognized. Hay and colleagues found that 30 percent of mothers of twins were depressed at three months postpartum ("What Information" 259). Choi et al. found 43 percent greater odds of moderate to severe depressive symptoms using the CES-D among mothers of twins at nine months postpartum (n=776) compared to singletons (n=7293). One qualitative study involving focus groups with twenty-nine mothers of multiples detailed the problem of depression (Ellison et al. 1426). Consistent with singleton research linking sleep deprivation with development of depression, both mothers quoted in Ellison's paper who reported postnatal depression also experienced severe sleep disturbance: "I told one of my neighbours, 'I've got to get somebody in here at night. I need to sleep'"; "I had postpartum depression. I was just a wreck. I couldn't handle it"; "I never got enough sleep. I became depressed and thought about suicide. Now I'm on antidepressants" (Ellison and Hall 411).

Increased risk of depression among mothers of multiples persisting well beyond the postnatal period is well documented. Thorpe and colleagues found that mothers of five-year-old twins were significantly more likely to be depressed than mothers of singletons (34.4 percent versus 22.5 percent). This finding was particularly informative because data were from the "pre-IVF" era and thus provide the clearest available picture of the direct impact of multiple birth on maternal mental health, without confounding by experiences of infertility and ART.

Rates among mothers of triplets are even greater, with clinical depression affecting 40 percent four months postpartum (Robin, Cahen, and Pons 1), and 25 percent being prescribed antidepressant medication at twelve months. All mothers of triplets in Garel and Blondel's study were significantly distressed at twelve months, and when followed up at four years, 36 percent were still depressed (Garel, Salobir, and Blondel 1162). Among Canadian mothers of twins and triplets, 42 percent had experienced postnatal depression, and 35 percent reported very high current levels of emotional stress (Parents of Multiple Births Association of Canada [POMBA])

Table One
Factors significantly associated with antenatal and postnatal depression
and with elevated risk among mothers of multiples

Risk factor	Antenatal Depression	Postnatal Depression	Elevated risk in multiple birth
Anxiety	✓	✓	Yes[b]
Life stress	✓[a]	✓	Yes[c]
Previous psychiatric illness	✓	✓	No
Lack of social support	✓[a]	✓	Yes[d]
Domestic violence	✓[a]		Unknown; plausible
Unintended pregnancy	✓		No[e]
Relationship factors	✓	✓	Yes[f]

Sources: after Scottish Intercollegiate Guidelines Network and (b) Nishihara et al.; Hay et al. "What information"; (c) Glazebrook et al.; Oliviennes et al.; (d) Baor and Soskolne; (f) Hay et al., ibid; McKay.

(a) Note: life stress, lack of social support and domestic violence remained significantly associated with depression on multivariate analysis.
Unplanned pregnancy is *less* likely among mothers of twins (due to prevalence of ART). However, for many women diagnosed with multiple pregnancy, reactions of shock and distress (Reinheckel et al.; Bryan, "Psychological Aspects"; Spillman) may parallel those associated with unintended pregnancy.

(Leonard 330). In a qualitative study involving nineteen mothers and fathers of multiple birth children, Reinheckel and colleagues concluded that the special problems of multiple parenthood (such as social isolation, marital and psychological problems) are not limited to higher order multiples or children with special needs, but that regardless of number of children, "Caring for the babies [leads] to the limits of parent's ability to take stress" (55). Raising multiples is difficult, even when the children are healthy, and insufficient social support predicts stress among mothers of twins (Baor and Soskolne 260).

MOTHERS OF MULTIPLES AND ANXIETY

Hay and colleagues found that 42 percent of mothers of three-month-old twins had high anxiety, three times the rate among mothers of singletons (Hay et al. 259). A more recent questionnaire study in western Japan that compared 119 mothers of twins aged from birth to two years old (recruited from twin support groups) and 109 mothers of singletons (from preschools and public health services) found significantly higher maternal anxiety among mothers of multiples. Parenting anxiety—including elevated "general confusion of parenting" and negative feelings towards their children—was related to delays in the children's development and was interpreted as evidence that compromised maternal mental health is detrimental to children (Nishihara et al. 831). Although this may be true, the alternative explanation that maternal anxiety may *result from* developmental delay in one or both twins was not offered.

CRITICISMS OF THE MEDICAL MODEL
OF POSTNATAL DEPRESSION

From adolescence to midlife, including during the reproductive life phase, women experience depression and anxiety at two to three times the rates experienced by men (Astbury 2; Fisher et al. "Women's Mental Health" 354). Feminist authors have argued that the medical model of postnatal depression neglects the heavily gendered social context in which mothering takes place, fails to acknowledge the emotional impact of a major life transition (Emmanuel and St John 2104), and emphasizes individual pathology while neglecting context and circumstances (Westall and Liamputtong 23).

Oates and colleagues conducted a qualitative study querying the universality of "postnatal depression" and regional attributions and beliefs regarding help for postnatally depressed mothers. Data were collected from fifteen sites in eleven countries, including Uganda, Portugal, and Japan. Participants were mothers of infants aged five to seven months (who participated in focus groups), fathers and grandmothers (who were interviewed individually), and health professionals. Morbid postnatal unhappiness was observed in all settings, and common causes were reported. Unhappiness following birth was attributed to loneliness, lack of emotional and practical social support, poor relationships with partners, family conflict, and tiredness. Mothers who were happy following birth had good social support. This study demonstrated that perception of postnatal unhappiness as an illness, requiring health intervention, was not universal. Appropriate assistance for postnatal unhappiness was suggested to include acceptance, understanding, and social support from family and social networks, and "talking therapies." Only in the United States was medication suggested as first-line management.

AN ALTERNATIVE CONCEPTUAL FRAMEWORK:
THE SOCIAL MODEL OF MENTAL HEALTH

The social model of health presumes that an individual's state of mental health (or experience of illness) is determined by personal experiences, social circumstances, culture, and political environment in addition to inherited or biological factors (Fisher, Rahman, Cabral de Mello, Chandra, and Herrman 432). As an alternative to the medical model of postnatal depression, the social theory of depression in women identifies personal loss, humiliation (an event rendering a person devalued in relation to others or self) and perceived entrapment as important precursors to depressive symptoms (Brown, Harris, and Hepworth 7). Fisher and colleagues argued that such experiences are particularly salient for new mothers (Fisher, Wynter, and

Rowe 432). A woman who becomes a mother loses previously valued roles (such as "worker" or "romantic partner") for a role that is relatively devalued. A responsive and interactive infant who feeds and settles well "rewards" his or her mother, whereas an infant who resists soothing or is difficult to feed may be experienced as critical of her efforts, a potential humiliation. The work of mothering a young infant is never "complete" and can be experienced as entrapment. Both poor self-efficacy and inadequate social support are plausibly linked to the notions of loss, humiliation, and entrapment. That circumstances of role loss, unsettled or crying infant/s, and endless uncompleted tasks are more frequently (and more intensely) experienced by mothers of multiples may explain elevated levels of distress.

Losses that are not, or cannot be, openly acknowledged, publicly mourned, or socially supported are known as "disenfranchised losses" (Doka 1). The losses associated with new motherhood (such as loss of autonomy or personal freedom) are disenfranchised losses. In the case of the new mother, these losses are not acknowledged by the community, as they are perceived as being inevitable consequences of becoming a mother. Mothers' feelings of shame for having negative feelings (in the context of performing a social role that is meant to be fulfilling) may exacerbate disenfranchised loss. According to the social model of postnatal mental health, features such as ambivalence towards the infant or feelings of inadequacy as a mother are not considered pathological but are instead viewed as understandable responses to a major life transition.

For all the personal gains that may accompany mothering multiples, there are many potential disenfranchised losses. A woman conceiving twins through IVF may fear expressing ambivalence, lest she be seen as "ungrateful." A first-time mother of twins may experience lingering sorrow that she was denied the opportunity to parent a "single baby" but cannot complain because she has an "instant family." A mother of multiples who wishes, but cannot afford, to return to paid work risks censure, should she complain about the dubious "luxury" of being a primary caregiver for multiples. Often, mothers' distress manifests as feelings of guilt over their own perceived inadequacies; they fear that they are failing to meet their children's competing needs as well as their own and others' expectations while they perform the work of mothering multiple children.

Consistent with the social model of health, researchers and policymakers are now describing "perinatal distress" to encompass depression, anxiety, and emotional adjustments rather than a distinct category entity of "postnatal depression" (McDonald et al. 316). The social model conceptualizes perinatal distress as a continuum from "no distress" to "extreme distress" on which an individual's position can change. This framework is more likely to capture the experience of mothering multiples than the medical model, as it acknowledges the relevance of the woman's social circumstances to her suffering rather than factors intrinsic to her individual character.

CONCLUSION

Poor maternal quality of life, parenting stress, and mental ill health are *not* the inevitable consequences of multiple birth. They may, however, be the inevitable consequences of *inadequately supported* multiple birth, which is widespread. When the risk and protective factors for mental health are considered, it is not surprising that outcomes for mothers of multiples can be poor. As a group, they experience multiple risks, including potentially traumatic pregnancy, birth, and perinatal period; special needs in one or more children; unsettled infants; fatigue; financial strain; compromised body image; diminished sense of competence; social isolation; and stigma. They have less access to protective factors, including adequate rest, time to pursue personal goals, companionship with partners and peers, and circumstance-specific information. Mothers can lack validation of their efforts, and may even face criticism—for example, assertions from attachment theorists that their mothering is inadequate compared to a singleton norm and is potentially damaging in failing to provide ample one-to-one interaction for each child. These messages can be internalized and induce feelings of guilt and inadequacy. Underpinning these is the pervasive cultural assumption that caregiving is a woman's responsibility and that it should be provided sensitively, effectively, alone, unremunerated, and without complaint. Gender considerations aside, it is questionable whether a single person can possibly meet the needs of two (or more) dependent children. Disproportionate distress and poor quality of life among mothers of multiples do not arise because mothers are "sick" or do not value their children, but because they are inadequately supported in the relentless performance of an often overwhelming task and are parenting in a social context that can be hostile. We argue that significant subjective maternal distress is an understandable response to what is frequently a highly distressing predicament.

Although this conclusion may appear pessimistic, there is good reason for optimism. Many of the challenges facing mothers of multiples are modifiable. However, solutions depend on shared responsibility and review of cultural norms and established theories. Recognition is a crucial first step. Even distress associated with non-modifiable adverse circumstances, such as a child's special needs, may respond to enhanced supportive interventions. The optimal solution is to prevent distress through universal initiatives rather than providing "treatment" when the problems are established. After a prolonged labour, it is possible to imagine the birth of a positive era, in which the exceptional circumstances of multiple birth are understood, accommodated, supported, and celebrated.

WORKS CITED

Abbink, C., et al. "Bonding as Perceived by Mothers of Twins." *Pediatric Nursing* 8.6 (1982): 411-413. Print.

Adams, S. S., et al. "Mode of Delivery and Postpartum Emotional Distress: A Cohort Study of 55,814 Women." *British Journal of Obstetrics and Gynaecology* 119.3 (2012): 298-305. Print.

Ainsworth, M. D. S., et al. *Patterns of Attachment: A Psychological Study of the Strange Situation.* Hillsdale: Erlbaum, 1978. Print.

Allen, E. C., et al. "Perception of Child Vulnerability among Mothers of Former Premature Infants." *Pediatrics* 113.2 (2004): 267-273. Print.

American Psychiatric Association. *Diagnostic and Statistical Manual of Mental Disorders DSM-IV TR (Text Revision).* Arlington: American Psychiatric Association, 2000. Print.

American Psychiatric Association. *Diagnostic and Statistical*

Manual of Mental Disorders, 5th Edition (DSM-5). Washington: American Psychiatric Association, 2013: 150. Print.

American Thoracic Society. "Statement on the Care of the Child with Chronic Lung Disease of Infancy and Childhood." *American Journal of Respiratory and Critical Care Medicine* 168 (2003): 356-396. Print.

"Are You Freaking out About Having Twins? You're Not Alone." *Sleeping Should Be Easy*, Nina, 2012. Web. 12 January 2015.

Armstrong, K. L., et al. "Sleep Deprivation or Postnatal Depression in Later Infancy: Separating the Chicken from the Egg." *Journal Of Paediatrics And Child Health* 34.3 (1998): 260-62. Print.

Astbury, J. *Gender Disparities in Mental Health*: Geneva: World Health Organization, 2001. Print.

Athanassiou, C. "A Study of the Vicissitudes of Identification in Twins." *International Journal of Psychoanalysis* 67 Part 3 (1986): 329-335. Print.

Australian Human Rights Commission (AHRC). "Balancing Paid Work and Family Responsibilities." AHRC, 2015. Web. 10 January 2015.

Australian Medical Association (AMA). *AMA Position Statement on Body Image and Health*, 2009. Print.

Australian Multiple Birth Association (ASMA). "Home Page." ASMA, 2012. Web. 18 February 2012.

Baor, L., and I. Blickstein. "En Route to an 'Instant Family'": Psychosocial Considerations." *Obstetric and Gynecological Clinics of North America* 32.1 (2005): 127-139. Print.

Baor, L., and V. Soskolne. "Mothers of IVF Twins: The Mediating Role of Employment and Social Coping Resources in Maternal Stress." *Women & Health* 52.3 (2012): 2522-64. Print.

Barclay, L., et al. "Becoming a Mother—An Analysis of Women's Experience of Early Motherhood." *Journal of Advanced Nursing* 25.4 (1997): 719-728. Print.

Barclay, L., and B. Lloyd. "The Misery of Motherhood: Alternative Approaches to Maternal Distress." *Midwifery* 12 (1996): 136-139. Print.

Barrett, Jon F. R., et al. "A Randomized Trial of Planned Cesarean or Vaginal Delivery for Twin Pregnancy." *New England Journal of Medicine* 369.14 (2013): 1295-1305. Print.

Barton, M. E., and R. Strosberg. "Conversational Patterns of Two-Year-Old Twins in Mother-Twin-Twin Triads." *Journal of Child Language* 24.1 (1997): 257-269. Print.

Bigelow, C., and J. Stone. "Bed Rest in Pregnancy." *Mount Sinai Journal of Medicine: A Journal of Translational and Personalized Medicine* 78.2 (2011): 291-302. Print.

Billings, J. "Bonding Theory—Tying Mothers in Knots? A Critical Review of the Application of a Theory to Nursing." *Journal of Clinical Nursing* 4 (1995): 207-211. Print.

Black, B. P., D. Holditch-Davis, and M. S. Miles. "Life Course Theory as a Framework to Examine Becoming a Mother of a Medically Fragile Preterm Infant." *Research in Nursing & Health* 32.1 (2009): 38-49. Print.

Bolch, C. E., et al. "Multiple Birth Families with Children with Special Needs: A Qualitative Investigation of Mothers' Experiences." *Twin Research and Human Genetics* 15.4 (2012): 503-515. Print.

Bolch, C. E., et al. "The MultiQOL Study: A Cross-Sectional Community Survey of Quality of Life Concerns of Parents of Young Multiple Birth Children in Australia." *Twins 2014: 15th Congress of the International Society of Twin Studies*. Ed. International Society of Twin Studies, 2014. 418-419. Print.

Bordo, S. *Unbearable Weight: Feminism, Western Culture, and the Body*. Berkeley: University of California Press, 1993. Print.

Bowlby, J. *Child Care and the Growth of Love*. Baltimore: Pelican Books, 1953. Print.

Bowman, K., and L. Ryan. *Twins: A Practical Guide to Parenting Multiples from Conception to Preschool*. Second ed. Crows Nest: Allen & Unwin, 2005. Print.

Brown, G. W., T. O. Harris, and C. Hepworth. "Loss, Humiliation and Entrapment among Women Developing Depression: A Patient and Non-Patient Comparison." *Psychological Medicine* 25.1 (1995): 7-21. Print.

Bryan, E. "Psychological Aspects of Prenatal Diagnosis and Its Implications in Multiple Pregnancies." *Prenatal Diagnosis* 25.9 (2005): 827-834. Print.

Bryan, E. "The Impact of Multiple Preterm Births on the Family." *BJOG: An International Journal of Obstetrics & Gynaecology*

110 (2003): 24-28. Print.

Campbell, D. M., and A. Templeton. "Maternal Complications of Twin Pregnancy." *International Journal of Gynaecology and Obstetrics* 84.1 (2004): 71-73. Print.

Chambers, P. L., E. M. Mahabee-Gittens, and A. C. Leonard. "Vulnerable Child Syndrome, Parental Perception of Child Vulnerability, and Emergency Department Usage." *Pediatric Emergency Care* 27.11 (2011): 1009-1013. Print.

Chang, C. "Raising Twin Babies and Problems in the Family." *Acta Geneticae Medicae et Gemellologiae (Roma)* 39.4 (1990): 501-05. Print.

Chatterji, P., and S. Markowitz. "Family Leave after Childbirth and the Mental Health of New Mothers." *Journal of Mental Health Policy and Economics* 15.2 (2012): 61-76. Print.

Chien, L. Y., et al. "Improved Outcome of Preterm Infants When Delivered in Tertiary Care Centers." *Obstetrics and Gynecology* 98.2 (2001): 247-252. Print.

Choi, Y., D. Bishai, and C. S. Minkovitz. "Multiple Births Are a Risk Factor for Postpartum Maternal Depressive Symptoms." *Pediatrics* 123.4 (2009): 1147-1154. Print.

Colpin, H. L., and L. Vandemeulebroecke. "Parenting Stress and Psychosocial Well-Being among Parents with Twins Conceived Naturally or by Reproductive Technology." *Human Reproduction* 14 (1999): 3133-3137. Print.

Cook, R., S. Bradley, and S. Golombok. "A Preliminary Study of Parental Stress and Child Behavior in Families with Twins Conceived by in-Vitro Fertilization." *Human Reproduction* 13 (1998): 3244-3246. Print.

Cooklin, A. R., et al. "Employment Conditions and Maternal Postpartum Mental Health: Results from the Longitudinal Study of Australian Children." *Archives of Women's Mental Health* 14.3 (2011): 217-225. Print.

Crowther, C. A. and S. Han. *Hospitalisation and Bed Rest for Multiple Pregnancy*: Cochrane Database of Systematic Reviews, 2010. Print.

Damato, E. G., and C. Burant. "Sleep Patterns and Fatigue in Parents of Twins." *Journal of Obstetric, Gynecologic, & Neonatal Nursing* 37.6 (2008): 738-749. Print.

Dennis, C. L., and L. Ross. "Relationships among Infant Sleep Patterns, Maternal Fatigue, and Development of Depressive Symptomatology." *Birth* 32.3 (2005): 187-193. Print.

"Did Anyone Decide Not to Return to Work after Having Twins?" *Circle of Moms*. Pop Sugar, 2010. Web. 5 January 2015.

Doka, K., ed. *Disenfranchised Grief: Recognizing Hidden Sorrow*. New York: Lexington Books, 1989. Print.

Eells, T. D. "Attachment Theory and Psychotherapy Research." *Journal of Psychotherapy Practice and Research* 10.2 (2001): 132-35. Print.

Eiser, C., et al. "Parenting the Premature Infant: Balancing Vulnerability and Quality of Life." *Journal of Child Psychology and Psychiatry and Allied disciplines* 46.11 (2005): 1169-1177. Print.

Ellison, M. A., and J. E. Hall. "Social Stigma and Compounded Losses: Quality-of-Life Issues for Multiple-Birth Families." *Fertility and Sterility* 80.2 (2003): 405-414. Print.

Ellison, M. A., et al. "Psychosocial Risks Associated with Multiple Births Resulting from Assisted Reproduction." *Fertility and Sterility* 83.5 (2005): 1422-1428. Print.

Emmanuel, E. and W. St John. "Maternal Distress: A Concept Analysis." *Journal of Advanced Nursing* 66.9 (2010): 2104-2115. Print.

Fenwick, Jennifer, Lesley Barclay, and Virginia Schmied. "Craving Closeness: A Grounded Theory Analysis of Women's Experiences of Mothering in the Special Care Nursery." *Women and Birth* 21.2 (2008): 71-85. Print.

Fierro, P. P. "Is Having Twins the Same as Having Two Children Close in Age?" *About Health*, About. 2010. Web. 8 February 2012.

Fierro, P. P. "Top 10 Ways to Increase Your Chances of Having Twins." *About Health*, About. 2012. Web. 12 March 2012.

Findler, L., O. Taubman-Ben-Ari, and K. Jacob. "Internal and External Contributors to Maternal Mental Health and Marital Adaptation One Year after Birth: Comparisons of Mothers of Pre-Term and Full-Term Twins." *Women & Health* 46.4 (2007): 39-60. Print.

Fisher, J., J. Astbury, and A. Smith. "Adverse Psychological Impact of Operative Obstetric Interventions: A Prospective Longitudinal

Study." *Australian and New Zealand Journal of Psychiatry* 31.5 (1997): 728-738. Print.

Fisher, J. and A. Stocky. "Maternal Perinatal Mental Health and Multiple Births: Implications for Practice." *Twin Research* 6.6 (2003): 506-513. Print.

Fisher, J., H. Rowe, and K. Hammarberg. "Admissions for Early Parenting Difficulties among Women with Infants Conceived by Assisted Reproductive Technologies: A Prospective Cohort Study." *Fertility and Sterility* 97.6 (2012): 1410-1416. Print.

Fisher, J. R. W., et al., eds. *Women's Mental Health*. New York: Oxford University Press, 2014. Print.

Fisher, J. R. W., K. Wynter, and H. J. Rowe. "Innovative Psycho-Educational Program to Prevent Common Postpartum Mental Disorders in Primiparous Women: A Before and After Controlled Study." *BMC Public Health* 10 (2010): 432. Print.

Fisher, J. R. W., C. J. Feekery, and H. J. Rowe-Murray. "Nature, Severity and Correlates of Psychological Distress in Women Admitted to a Private Mother-Baby Unit." *Journal Of Paediatrics And Child Health* 38.2 (2002): 140-145. Print.

Fisher, J., et al. "Mental Health of Parents and Infant Health and Development in Resource-Constrained Settings: Evidence Gaps and Implications for Facilitating 'Good-Enough Parenting' in the Twenty-First-Century World." *Parenthood and Mental Health: A Bridge between Infant and Adult Psychiatry*. Eds. Tyano, S., et al. London: John Wiley & Sons, Ltd., 2010. 429-442. Print.

Gallo, A-M., and K. A. Lee. "Sleep Characteristics in Hospitalized Antepartum Patients." *Journal of Obstetric, Gynecologic, & Neonatal Nursing* 37.6 (2008): 715-721. Print.

Garel, M., C. Salobir, and B. Blondel. "4 Year Follow-up of Mothers of Triplets." *Fertility and Sterility* 67 (1997): 1162-1165. Print.

Garel, M., and B. Blondel. "Assessment at 1 Year of the Psychological Consequences of Having Triplets." *Human Reproduction* 7.5 (1992): 729-732. Print.

Garel, M., E. Charlemaine, and S. Missonnier. "Multiple Fetuses Pregnancy and Other Medical High-Risk Pregnancies." *Parenthood and Mental Health: A Bridge between Infant and Adult Psychiatry*. Eds. Tyano, S., et al. London: John Wiley & Sons, Ltd., 2010. 99-107. Print.

Giallo, R., et al. "Assessment of Maternal Fatigue and Depression in the Postpartum Period: Support for Two Separate Constructs." *Journal of Reproductive and Infant Psychology* 29.1 (2011): 69-80. Print.

Gjerdingen, D., et al. "Predictors of Mothers' Postpartum Body Dissatisfaction." *Women & Health* 49.6 (2009): 491-504. Print.

Gjerdingen, D. K., and B. P. Yawn. "Postpartum Depression Screening: Importance, Methods, Barriers, and Recommendations for Practice." *Journal of the American Board of Family Medicine* 20.3 (2007): 280-288. Print.

Glazebrook, C., et al. "Parenting Stress in First-Time Mothers of Twins and Triplets Conceived after in Vitro Fertilization." *Fertility and Sterility* 81.3 (2004): 505-511. Print.

Gromada, K. K., and M. C. Hurlburt. *Keys to Parenting Multiples.* Second ed. New York: Barron's, 2001. Print.

Gross, D., and L. Rocissano. "Maternal Confidence in Toddlerhood: Its Measurement for Clinical Practice and Research." *Nurse Practitioner* 13 (1988): 19-29. Print.

Gupton, R. N., M. Heaman, and L. W. Cheung. "Complicated and Uncomplicated Pregnancies: Women's Perception of Risk." *Journal of Obstetric, Gynecologic, & Neonatal Nursing* 30.2 (2001): 192-201. Print.

Guzman-Marin, R., et al. "Hippocampal Neurogenesis Is Reduced by Sleep Fragmentation in the Adult Rat." *Neuroscience* 148 (2007): 325-333. Print.

"Gymboree—Not Possible with 18 mo .Twins?" *Babycenter Community*. BabyCenter, 2012. Web. 20 July 2012.

"Hardest Part About Having Twins" *Babycenter* Community. BabyCenter, 17 November 2010. Web. 1 September 2012.

"Having Twins and Triplets—Interesting and Fun Facts." *Twins UK*. Twins International Ltd., 2012. Web. 12 March 2012.

Hay, D. A. "Adolescent Twins and Secondary Schooling." *Twin and Triplet Psychology: A Professional Guide to Working with Multiples*. Ed. Sandbank, A. London and New York: Routledge, 1999. 119-142. Print.

Hay, D. A., et al. "What Information Should the Multiple Birth Family Receive before, During and after the Birth?" *Acta Geneticae Medicae et Gemellologiae (Roma)* 39.2 (1990): 259-269. Print.

Hay, D. A., et al. "Twin Children in Volunteer Registries: Biases in Parental Participation and Reporting." *Acta Geneticae Medicae et Gemellologiae (Roma)* 39.1 (1990): 71-84. Print.

Hay, D. A., and P. J. O'Brien. "Early Influences on the School Social Adjustment of Twins." *Acta Geneticae Medicae et Gemellologiae (Roma)* 36 (1987): 239-248. Print.

Holditch-Davis, D., D. Roberts, and M. Sandelowski. "Early Parental Interactions with and Perceptions of Multiple Birth Infants." *Journal of Advanced Nursing* 30.1 (1999): 200-210. Print.

Hübner-Liebermann, B., H. Hausner, and M. Wittmann. "Recognizing and Treating Peripartum Depression." *Deutsches Ärzteblatt International* 109.24 (2012): 419. Print.

"I Hate My Belly after Twins" *Raising Twins*. Weblog, 2012. 6 January 2015

"'I Would Love to Have Twins!!'" *Circle of Moms*. Pop Sugar, 2009. Web. 13 February 2012

Irish Mutiple Birth Association (IMBA). "Home Page of Irish Multiple Birth Association." IMBA, 2015. Web. 3 July 2015.

"IVF or Natural—Why Do People Think They Have a Right to Know?" *Circle of Moms*. Pop Sugar, 2009. Web. 5 January 2015.

Kessler, R. C., K. D. Mickelson, and D. R. Williams. "The Prevalence, Distribution, and Mental Health Correlates of Perceived Discrimination in the United States." *Journal of Health and Social Behavior* 40.3 (1999): 208-230. Print.

Kulkarni, A. D., et al. "Fertility Treatments and Multiple Births in the United States." *New England Journal of Medicine* 369.23 (2013): 2218-2225. Print.

Leahy-Warren, P., G. McCarthy, and P. Corcoran. "First-Time Mothers: Social Support, Maternal Parental Self-Efficacy and Postnatal Depression." *Journal of Clinical Nursing* 21.3-4 (2012): 388-397. Print.

Lee, S. Y., and K. A. Lee. "Early Postpartum Sleep and Fatigue for Mothers after Cesarean Delivery Compared with Vaginal Delivery: An Exploratory Study." *Journal of Perinatal and Neonatal Nursing* 21.2 (2007): 109-113. Print.

Lenz, E. R., et al. "The Middle-Range Theory of Unpleasant Symptoms: An Update." *Advances in Nursing Science* 19.3 (1997): 14-27. Print.

Leonard, Linda G. "Depression and Anxiety Disorders During Multiple Pregnancy and Parenthood." *Journal of Obstetric, Gynecologic, & Neonatal Nursing* 27.3 (1998): 329-337. Print.

Li, Z., et al. *Australia's Mothers and Babies 2011.* Canberra: AIHW, 2013. Print.

Luke, B. "Nutrition in Multiple Gestations." *Clinics in Perinatology* 32.2 (2005): 403-429. Print.

Lupton, D., and J. Fenwick. "'They've Forgotten That I'm the Mum': Constructing and Practising Motherhood in Special Care Nurseries." *Social Science and Medicine* 53.8 (2001): 1011-1021. Print.

Maloni, J. A. "Astronauts & Pregnancy Bed Rest." *AWHONN Lifelines* 6.4 (2002): 318-323. Print.

Maloni, J. A., Seunghee Park Margevicius, and Elizabeth G. Damato. "Multiple Gestation: Side Effects of Antepartum Bed Rest." *Biological Research For Nursing* 8.2 (2006): 115-128. Print.

Maslow, A. H. "A Theory of Human Motivation." *Psychological Review* 50.4 (1943): 370-396. Print.

McDonald, S., et al. "Development of a Prenatal Psychosocial Screening Tool for Post-Partum Depression and Anxiety." *Paediatric Perinatal Epidemiology* 26.4 (2012): 316-327. Print.

McKay, S. *The Effects of Twins and Multiple Births on Families and Their Living Standards.* Birmingham: University of Birmingham, 2010. Print.

McLeod, S. A. "John Bowlby: Maternal Deprivation Theory." *Simply Psychology.* N.p., 2007. Web. 12 May 2012.

Meerlo, P., et al. "New Neurons in the Adult Brain: The Role of Sleep and Consequences of Sleep Loss." *Sleep Medicine Review* 13.3 (2009): 187-194. Print.

Megel, M. E., et al. "Baby Lost and Found: Mothers' Experiences of Infants Who Cry Persistently." *Journal of Pediatric Health Care* 25.3 (2011): 144-152. Print.

"Mothers Group, Is It Worth It?" *Essential Baby,* 31 January 2006. Web. 3 May 2012.

Multiples of America. "Home Page of Multiples of America." Multiples of America, 2015. Web. 3 July 2015.

Narvaez, D. "Dangers of 'Crying It Out': Damaging Children and Their Relationships for the Longterm." *Psychology Today.*

Sussex Publishers, 2011. Web. 12 January 2015.

Neifert, M., and J. Thorpe. "Twins: Family Adjustment, Parenting, and Infant Feeding in the Fourth Trimester." *Clinical Obstetrics and Gynecology* 33.1 (1990): 102-113. Print.

Nettleton, Sarah. *The Sociology of Health and Fitness.* Cambridge: Polity Press, 2006. Print.

Nishihara, R., et al. "Parenting Anxiety and Childhood Development of Twins as Compared to Singletons." *Nippon Koshu Eisei Zasshi* 53.11 (2006): 831-841. Print.

Noble, R. E. "Depression in Women." *Metabolism: Clinical and Experimental* 54.5 (2005): 49-52. Print.

Novati, A., et al. "Chronic Sleep Restriction Causes a Decrease in Hippocampal Volume in Adolescent Rats, Which Is Not Explained by Changes in Glucocorticoid Levels or Neurogenesis." *Neuroscience* 190 (2011): 145-155. Print.

Nys, K., et al. "Feelings and the Need for Information and Counselling of Expectant Parents of Twins." *Twin Research* 1.3 (1998): 142-149. Print.

O'Brien, E. T., S. Quenby, and T. Lavender. "Women's Views of High Risk Pregnancy under Threat of Preterm Birth." *Sexual and Reproductive Healthcare* 1.3 (2010): 79-84. Print.

Oates, M. R., et al. "Postnatal Depression across Countries and Cultures: A Qualitative Study." *British Journal of Psychiatry Supplement* 184.16 (2004): s10-16. Print.

Olivennes, F., et al. "Behavioral and Cognitive Development as Well as Family Functioning of Twins Conceived by Assisted Reproduction: Findings from a Large Population Study." *Fertility and Sterility* 84.3 (2005): 725-733. Print.

"Parents Group." *Essential Baby*, 14 July 2009. Web. 3 March 2012.

Phares, V. "Where's Poppa? The Relative Lack of Attention to the Role of Fathers in Child and Adolescent Psychopathology." *American Psychologist* 47 (1992): 656-664. Print.

"Pigeon Pair." *Weblog.* Weblog, 2010. Web. 12 March 2012.

Pinar, H., et al. "Reference Values for Singleton and Twin Placental Weights." *Pediatr Pathol Lab Med* 16.6 (1996): 901-907. Print.

Post and Antenatal Depression Association. "What Is Postnatal Depression? Fact Sheet 14." Melbourne: Post and Antenatal

Depression Association Inc., 2012. Print.

"Practical Help and Financial Factsheet for Families with Twins, Triplets or More." *Twins UK*. Twins International Ltd., 2015. Web. 3 July 2015.

"Pregnant for the First Time with Twins ...What Should I Expect?" *Circle of Moms*. Pop Sugar, 2009. Web. 3 November 2011.

Raj, S. and R. Morley. "'Are You Asking Me If We Had Sex to Conceive?' To Whom Do Parents of Twins Disclose Mode of Conception and What Do They Feel About Being Asked?" *Twin Research and Human Genetics* 10.6 (2007): 886-891. Print.

Rasmussen, K. M., A. L. Yaktine, and Committee to Reexamine IOM Pregnancy Weight Guidelines. *Weight Gain During Pregnancy: Reexamining the Guidelines*: Institute of Medicine, National Research Council, 2009. Print.

Reinheckel, A., et al. "[Life Situation of Parents of Twins and Triplets: A Qualitative Study].[Article in German]." *Zeitschrift fur Geburtshilfe und Neonatologie* 204.2 (2000): 55-59. Print.

Riemann, D., and U. Voderholzer. "Primary Insomnia: A Risk Factor to Develop Depression?" *Journal of Affective Disorders* 76 (2003): 255-259. Print.

Robin, M., D. Corroyer, and I. Casati. "Childcare Patterns of Mothers of Twins During the First Year." *Journal of Child Psychology and Psychiatry* 37.4 (1996): 453-460. Print.

Robin, M., D. Josse, and C. Tourrette. "Mother-Twin Interaction During Early Childhood." *Acta Geneticae Medicae et Gemellologiae (Roma)* 37.2 (1988): 151-159. Print.

Robin, M., F. Cahen, and J. C. Pons. "Maternal Adjustment to a Multiple Birth." *Early Child Development and Care* 79.1 (1992): 1-11. Print.

Roca-de Bes, M., J. Gutierrez-Maldonado, and J. M. Gris-Martínez. "Comparative Study of the Psychosocial Risks Associated with Families with Multiple Births Resulting from Assisted Reproductive Technology (Art) and without Art." *Fertility and Sterility* 96.1 (2011): 170-174. Print.

Ross, L. E., B. J. Murray, and M. Steiner. "Sleep and Perinatal Mood Disorders: A Critical Review." *Journal of Psychiatry and Neuroscience* 30.4 (2005): 247-256. Print.

Rothbaum, F., et al. "Attachment and Culture. Security in the

United States and Japan." *The American Psychologist* 55.10 (2000): 1092-1104. Print.

Roudsari, B. S., et al. "Risk of Early Childhood Injuries in Twins and Singletons." *Journal of Early Childhood Research* 4.2 (2006): 121-131. Print.

Rowe-Murray, H. J., and J. R. W. Fisher. "Operative Intervention in Delivery Is Associated with Compromised Early Mother-Infant Interaction." *BJOG: An International Journal of Obstetrics & Gynaecology* 108.10 (2001): 1068-1075. Print.

Rubarth, L. B., et al. "Women's Experience of Hospitalized Bed Rest During High-Risk Pregnancy." *Journal of Obstetric, Gynecologic, & Neonatal Nursing* 41.3 (2012): 398-407. Print.

Ruiz, R. J., C. E. L. Brown, and P. A. Kirk. "The Research Basis for Prevention of Preterm Delivery in Twin Gestations." *Online Journal of Knowledge Synthesis for Nursing* E5.1 (1998): 15-27. Print.

Sandbank, A. "Personality, Identity and Family Relationships." *Twin and Triplet Psychology: A Professional Guide to Working with Multiples.* Ed. A. Sandbank. New York: Routledge, 1999. Print.

Scottish Intercollegiate Guidelines Network (SIGN). *Management of Perinatal Mood Disorders.* Edinburgh: SIGN, 2012. Print.

Singer, L. T., et al. "Longitudinal Predictors of Maternal Stress and Coping after Very Low-Birth-Weight Birth." *Archives of Pediatric and Adolescent Medicine* 164.6 (2010): 518-524. Print.

Sit, D., A. J. Rothschild, and K. L. Wisner. "A Review of Postpartum Psychosis." *Journal of Women's Health (Larchmont)* 15.4 (2006): 352-368. Print.

Sosa, C., et al. *Bed Rest in Singleton Pregnancies for Preventing Preterm Birth*: Cochrane Database of Systematic Reviews, 2010. Print.

Spillman, J. R. "'You Have a Little Bonus, My Dear'. The Effect on Mothers of the Diagnosis of a Multiple Pregnancy." *British Medical Ultrasound Society Bulletin* 39 (1985): 6-9. Print.

Stahl, K., and V. Hundley. "Risk and Risk Assessment in Pregnancy—Do We Scare Because We Care?" *Midwifery* 19.4 (2003): 298-309. Print.

Stramrood, C. A., et al. "Posttraumatic Stress Following Childbirth in Homelike - and Hospital Settings." *Journal of Psychosomatic Obstetrics & Gynecology* 32.2 (2011): 88-97. Print.

Studd, J., and R. E. Nappi. "Reproductive Depression." *Gynecology and Endocrinology* 28.Supplement 1 (2012): 42-45. Print.

Swanson, L. M., et al. "Relationships among Depression, Anxiety, and Insomnia Symptoms in Perinatal Women Seeking Mental Health Treatment." *Journal of Women's Health* 20.4 (2011): 553-558. Print.

The Royal Australian and New Zealand College of Obstetricians and Gynaecologists. "Caesarean Delivery on Maternal Request (Cdmr)." Ed. The Royal Australian and New Zealand College of Obstetricians and Gynaecologists, 2013. Print.

"Things Not to Say to a Twin Mum." *Weblog*. Weblog, 10 January 2012. Web. 5 May 2012.

Thomas, J. G. "The Early Parenting of Twins." *Military Medicine* 161.4 (1996): 233-235. Print.

Thorpe, K., R. Greenwood, and T. Goodenough. "Does a Twin Pregnancy Have a Greater Impact on Physical and Emotional Well-Being Than a Singleton Pregnancy?" *Birth* 22.3 (1995): 148-152. Print.

"Time for an Update." Australian Multiple Birth Association, 2009. Web. 29 September 2010.

Topiwala, A., G. Hothi, and K. P. Ebmeier. "Identifying Patients at Risk of Perinatal Mood Disorders." *Practitioner* 256.1751 (2012): 15-18. Print.

"Twin Mums Are Freaks of Nature." Weblog, 2010. Web. 8 February 2012.

"Which One Is the Aggressive One?" *Twin Pregnancy and Beyond*. N.p, 5 June 2011. Web. 4 March 2012.

Umstad, M. P., et al. "Multiple Deliveries: The Reduced Impact of in Vitro Fertilisation in Australia." *Aust N Z J Obstet Gynaecol* 53.2 (2013): 158-164. Print.

Vayssière, C., et al. "Twin Pregnancies: Guidelines for Clinical Practice from the French College of Gynaecologists and Obstetricians (Cngof)." *European Journal of Obstetrics and Gynecology and Reproductive Biology* 156.1 (2011): 12-17. Print.

Vigod, S. N., et al. "Prevalence and Risk Factors for Postpartum Depression among Women with Preterm and Low-Birth-Weight

Infants: A Systematic Review." *British Journal of Obstetrics and Gynaecology* 117.5 (2010): 540-550. Print.

Wandersman, L.P., A. Wandersman, and S. Kahn. "Social Support in the Transition to Parenthood." *Journal of Community Psychology* 8.4 (1980): 332-342. Print.

Westall, C. and P. Liamputtong. *Motherhood and Postnatal Depression: Narratives of Women and Their Partners.* Dordrecht, Heidelberg, London, & New York: Springer, 2011. Print.

"Subconscious Favouritism?" What to Expect Foundation, 2011. Web. 15 March 2012.

White, C. P., M. B. White, and M. A. Fox. "Maternal Fatigue and Its Relationship to the Caregiving Environment." *Families, Systems and Health* 27.4 (2009): 325-345. Print.

Workplace Fairness. "Family Responsibilities Discrimination." *Workplace Fairness*, 2010. Web. 10 January 2015.

Zheng, M. M., et al. "Comparison of Second-Trimester Maternal Serum Free-Beta-Human Chorionic Gonadotropin and Alpha-Fetoprotein between Normal Singleton and Twin Pregnancies: A Population-Based Study." *Chin Med J (Engl)* 123.5 (2010): 555-558. Print.

Visual Interlude I

curated by Kathy Mantas

2.
A Glimpse into a Multiple Birth Mother's Life

BONNIE L. SCHULTZ

ARTIST'S STATEMENT

FROM A WOMAN'S SOUL—THROUGH A WOMAN'S EYES—
BY A WOMAN'S HANDS

When I was a child, a blank sheet of paper was my creative space, open wide with possibility and invitation. My art, rigid and controlled, highly organized, and mostly realistic, evolved to be free, impressionistic, and colourful. Over the years, I have tried almost every craft, chalking it up to an intense curiosity that drives me and a strong, over-creative soul exploring ways to express itself. I have explored various materials and processes throughout the years. My art is influenced by everything that I see, feel, and experience, and I am inspired daily by my family, friends, and Mother Earth. It has been, and continues to be, an amazing life journey with no room for things that lack personal meaning or memories for me.

My multimedia art projects turn my joys and sorrows into a celebration of life and love, capturing moments in nature and life, often coupled with positive affirmations of love, hope, and inspiration. As a mother of twin girls and two singleton girls, life was hectic, disorganized, wonderful, precious, and exhausting—all at the same time! Laundry piled high, house upside down, and kids going in different directions. Their little hands stole my heart and their little feet ran away with it!

These playful, whimsical sketches look at the lighter side of multiple birth life, giving HOPE, a smile, and maybe even a chuckle or two to mothers (and fathers or parents) who are immersed in the daily routines of raising multiples. Everyone's story is different, filled with joy, hardships, loss, celebrations, special friendships, and lots and lots of love!

The sketches included here were created quickly on random bits of paper, simply due to constraints on my time as a mom of four young children all those years ago. They were originally created for Multiple Births Canada for use in their publications and quarterly magazine, *Multiple Moments*, but were never published. This series of sketches depict only a *small glimpse of life* for a mother of multiples—from finding out the news of the pregnancy, to seeing a little bump that soon becomes a big bump, to patiently awaiting the babies' arrival, and to sometimes being surprised that there are more than two!

Illustrated here are motherhood and its many possible stages: the laundry that never seems to end; thoughts of running away; the moment of waiting to hear their little voices (and then wanting them to stop!) Last, but not least, came the survival years of raising multiples through the toddler ages to teenagers, coping with the usual challenges as well as the unique issues of individuality, sibling rivalry, and multiples in school, to just name a few.

Yes, I am proudly a Mom ... and I enjoy trips to the bathroom alone, naps, and silence!

—Bonnie L. Schultz, Alberta, Canada

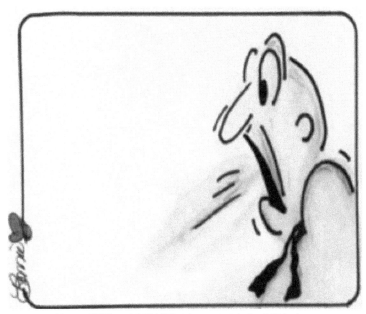

You are kidding, right!? 1986, Ink pen sketch, 5 x 3.25 inches

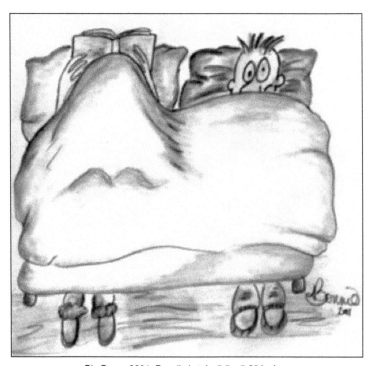

Big Bump, 2001, Pencil sketch, 5.5 x 5.25 inches

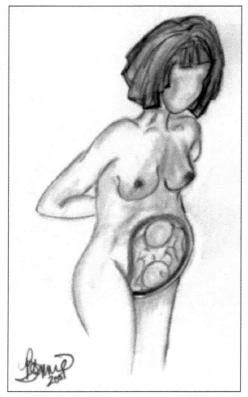

Are they here yet? 2001, Pencil sketch, 5 x 2.75 inches

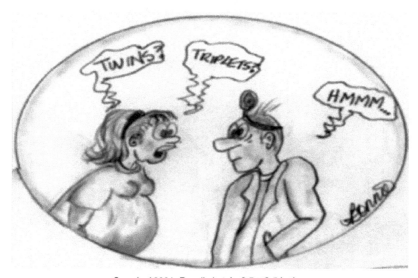

Surprise! 2001, Pencil sketch, 3.5 x 3.5 inches

I'm a Mom!

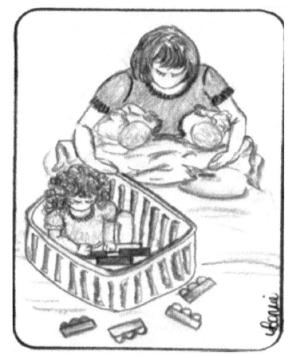

I Make Milk, 1994, Pencil sketch, 3.5 x 5.5 inches

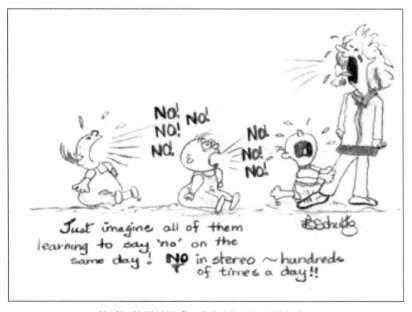

No, No, No!!! 1994, Pencil sketch, 5.5 x 4.75 inches

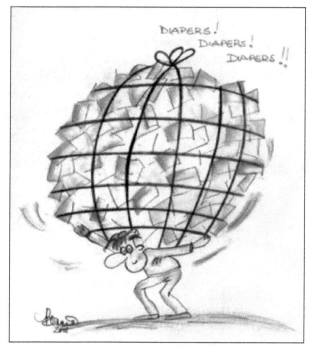

Too many diapers! 2001, Pencil sketch, 5.75 x 6.75 inches

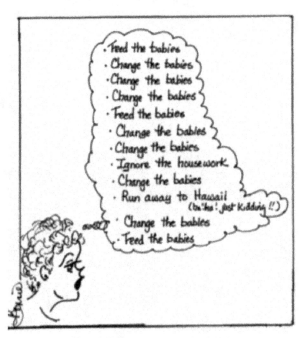

Hawaii, 1986, Ink pen, 5.75 x 6 inches

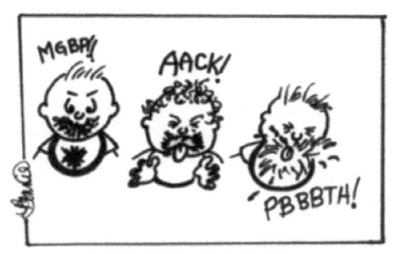

Get The Hose! 1990, Pencil sketch, 4.5 x 3.25 inches

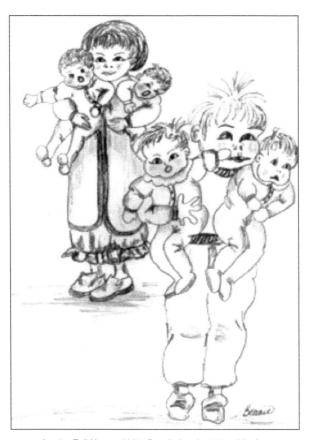

2 + 4 = Full House, 2001, Pencil sketch, 5.25 x 8 inches

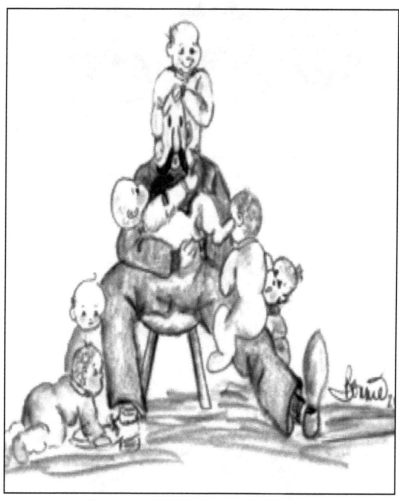

Mom's night out! 2001,Pencil sketch, 6.5 x 4.75 inches

You are one of the triplets?
But, which one are you???

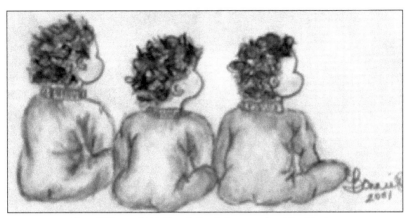

Same/Different, 2001, Pencil sketch & watercolor, 4.5 x 3 inches

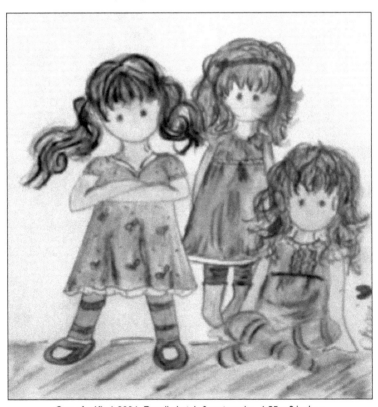

One of a Kind, 2004, Pencil sketch & watercolor, 4.25 x 6 inches

Mooooom!!!! He's touching me!!!

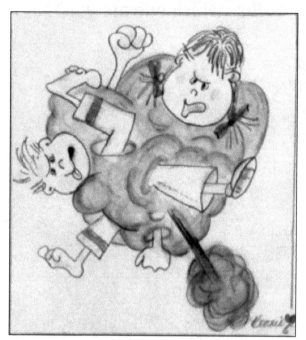

Sibling Love, 2009, Pencil sketch & watercolor, 4.5 x 4.76 inches

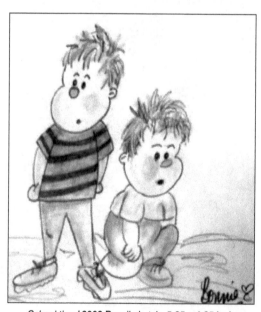

School time! 2002, Pencil sketch, 5.25 x 4.25 inches

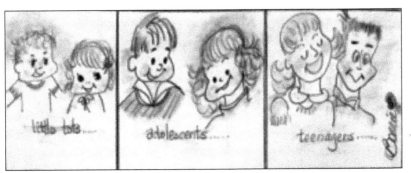

The Joy of Multiples! 2002, Pencil sketch, 2 x 5.75 inches

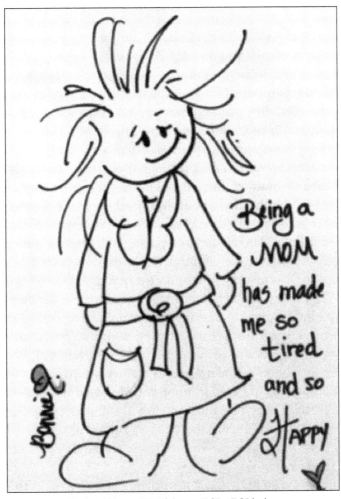

Tired and Happy, 2004, Ink pen, 5.25 x 7.25 inches

3.
You're So Lucky

SUZANNE KAMATA

I WAS AFRAID of the pain. Almost from the minute I knew I was pregnant with twins, I dreaded the trauma of childbirth. I could handle the three to five months of nausea, the insomnia, the weight gain, even the responsibilities of the next eighteen or so years, but not, I thought, the most agonizing pain known to womankind.

My sister-in-law in Ohio gave birth to a six pound twelve ounce boy in two hours with an epidural. "It was almost fun," she told me. "I could feel him coming through the birth canal, but it didn't hurt." She showed me the video—Elton John played on a boom box; her mother bustled about. My brother narrated the event.

"That's what I want, too," I said. Except instead of Elton John, we'd have Enya. There'd be champagne chilling in the mini-fridge. Of course, I'd have the epidural. My mother wouldn't be in the delivery room—just my husband, Yukiyoshi.

But I live in Japan and no one that I talked to here had ever heard of any kind of anaesthesia during normal childbirth. My friend Mariko, who gave birth to a nearly ten-pound baby, was in labour for twenty-four hours with no pain relief. In Japan, I'd heard a woman in labour was supposed to endure her pain in silence. If she cried out, she'd failed in some way. I vowed to be silent.

Even though they don't use anaesthesia, Japanese women have age-old ways of reducing the pain. A small baby makes for an easy delivery and several women gave me advice on restricting the size of my twins.

"You should go for walks," a mother of two told me. "You don't want the babies to get too big."

70

"Don't let your legs get cold," another woman advised. "Cold legs can lead to a miscarriage."

In my fifth month of pregnancy, my mother-in-law announced that it was time for an *obi*—a thick band tied around my waist to keep the babies from getting too large. I was horrified. It sounded worse than Chinese foot-binding. Twins are usually underweight, and I didn't want to do anything to impede their growth.

I asked my obstetrician about the practice, just to be polite. I had no intention of wrapping my middle.

"In the old days," he explained, "people had their babies at home. There was no recourse in the event of a difficult birth. They did whatever they could to have an easy labour."

I didn't go for walks. I lazed around on the sofa admiring baby clothes in the *Land's End* catalogue. I watched CNN and ABC news on satellite TV. I snuggled under an afghan, keeping my legs warm. And I threw up. And then I started to bleed.

I was hospitalized due to a threatened miscarriage. My room was across from the delivery room, and I could hear women screaming out in the night: "*Itai! Itai! Itai!*" ["It hurts! It hurts! It hurts!"], "*Iya! Iya! Iya!*" ["No! No! No!"]. I was terrified. I wondered if it was too late to change my mind.

The doctor recommended *cerclage*, a procedure in which the cervix is sutured shut to help prevent premature labour. After my first scare, he didn't have to work hard to persuade me.

"Do you want anaesthesia?" he asked me. "And if so, what kind?"

He told me that some women went through the operation with no pain relief at all. It sounded brave, but I am a wimp. "Give me the spinal," I said.

Before the operation, I was jabbed with a needle in the arm. When it was time for the epidural, I assumed the fetal pose and waited for the prick in my spine. In the United States, an anaesthesiologist would have handled this part, but there was no one extra in that Japanese hospital room, just the obstetrician and nurses. My mind was haunted by newspaper stories of mixed-up medicines and incompetent hospital doctors. If he missed, would I be paralysed for life?

I was nude, and everyone else was garbed in sterile blue, mouths hidden by ridged masks, only dark eyes visible. They didn't say anything except "This'll hurt." I wanted to ask someone to tell me a story, to distract me with words and questions like Dr. Raymond back in South Carolina.

I felt a cool hand pressing on my thigh, keeping me still for the needle that was about to go in. The first time, I flinched a little, but didn't make a sound. It didn't really hurt until the liquid was injected, and then it ached so much that I clenched my jaw.

I heard the doctor sigh. "Sorry. Gotta try it again."

It took two more jabs before the needle was properly inserted. Each time I felt the same ache, but I didn't cry out. Not even a whimper.

I borrowed videos on Lamaze from the hospital. The woman in the first video made it look so easy. She didn't scream, although a few tears trickled down her cheek. The baby slithered right out of her and was suddenly at her breast.

The Lamaze method: breathe in and breathe out with the pain. In, out. I practised. I thought that maybe it wouldn't be so bad after all.

I was surprised by blood again when I was six-months pregnant.

"Threatened premature labour," the doctor said, and he sent me to bed for the remaining three months of my pregnancy.

I was hooked up to an IV, and my movements were restricted. I brushed my teeth while on my back and ate my meals at a forty-five degree angle. For ten days, my feet did not touch the floor. Even so, my belly continued to tighten with contractions and blood stained the white sheets.

I was transferred by ambulance to another, bigger hospital—one with lots of incubators and a brand new Neonatal Intensive Care Unit (NICU). This time I had roommates: two other women who were expecting twins in July. Mine were due in September.

The other women were there according to hospital policy. Since there is an increased risk of premature labour for multiple pregnancies, women expecting more than one baby are put under observation as a matter of course in the eighth month.

We passed around magazines and brainstormed baby names. We traded snacks and old wives' tales. We worried together about the pain of childbirth. My second night there, we talked about ordering a pizza in a few days. It was like an adult slumber party.

A friend brought me novels. I read all day. Once in awhile, a nurse came to monitor the babies' heartbeats. They kicked and squirmed, and their hearts were strong.

My parents called each morning from South Carolina, and my mother-in-law dropped by with washed pyjamas and cream puffs. The aunt of my sister-in-law's husband came by along with a friend of my husband's family. "You shouldn't read," the aunt told me. "It excites the mind and is bad for your baby." She said that I should lie quietly and talk to my babies. For three months.

My husband came every day after teaching high school physical education classes and coaching baseball. He brought my mail.

I was starting to relax. I was even beginning to enjoy myself. The doctor announced that I could start using the toilet again. The catheter was removed, and I began testing my shaky legs, taking my first tentative steps toward wellness. Or so I thought.

The next morning, I awoke soaked in blood. My roommates slept through my frantic call to the nurse. Soon, I lay on an operating table awaiting an emergency C-section. I was surrounded by Japanese-speaking strangers, wearing blue gauze masks and matching smocks. Yukiyoshi was outside in a waiting room with my wedding ring in his pocket (no jewellery allowed during surgery). The rest of my family was thousands of miles away. I had lived in Japan for ten years, but it had never felt as foreign as it did at this moment.

"*Itai, itai, itai,*" I said. I'd gone through thirty minutes of labour and already my vow of silence was shattered. I was secretly impressed, however, by my ability to communicate in a foreign language in such extreme circumstances.

I'd expected everything to be different. I'd expected ice cubes in my mouth and my husband's fingers kneading my lower back. Instead, I was clutching the hand of a stranger, and I was scared.

Someone told me to curl up in a ball. I eased onto my side and curled. I felt the needle slide into my spine, but this time it didn't hurt at all. My lower body became warm and then went quickly numb.

The obstetrician started swabbing my middle with antiseptic. Another man, identified as the neonatal specialist, entered the room. "Twenty-six-weeks-old baby very difficult," he told me in heavily accented English. "I will do my best."

I looked at the clock. It was eight-thirty in the morning. I didn't want to think about what was going to happen in the hours, days, weeks to follow.

I was sorry that I'd ever wished for an easy birth. With a few extra weeks in the womb, my babies' lungs would have fully developed. They'd have enough fat on their bodies to maintain the proper temperature. They would have received vital antibodies and nutrients through the placenta. These gifts of the body made my fear of physical pain seem petty.

Minutes later, the obstetrician sliced open my abdomen and pulled out my son. I couldn't see what was happening because a screen had been set up over my chest, but I could feel the liquid ooze over my belly and the fish-like squirm of my 964-gram baby boy. "*Kawaii*," the nurse holding my hand said. "He's cute." I heard his cry, a tiny mewling, before he was whisked away.

"Now we'll go in for the other one," the doctor said. He quickly delivered my 690-gram daughter, the one who had lived beneath my heart for six and a half months. And then she was gone, too.

I lay on the table, resigned and passive. I had avoided the dreaded pain of pushing two babies through the birth canal—how lucky!—but I felt like a failure. Although I'd tried to do the right thing throughout—abstaining from coffee and alcohol, avoiding travel and smoky rooms—there was a chance that my babies wouldn't make it through the day.

Because I was recovering from surgery, I didn't see my children for twenty-four hours. My husband was allowed into the NICU and he reported back to me. "They're cute," he said, "but not like that." He pointed to the babies on the cover of one of my books. "They look like little baby birds."

Luckily, miraculously, my babies survived through the night. The following evening, I was wheeled to the NICU, and I saw my children for the first time. Their bodies were scrawny and red, but they had all ten fingers and toes. I couldn't see their eyes because they were fused shut. They had dark hair on their heads and soft hairs on their shoulders and faces. They both had little beards.

The neonatal specialist, Dr. Honda, was the man who was supposed to keep my children alive. When I first saw him, the word that popped into my head was "young." He had brush-cut hair and dimples. His ample belly strained against the pink smock. From the back, I could see that he was wearing a T-shirt underneath— casual clothes when professionalism would seem to dictate button downs and neckties. Get my babies out of here, I thought. I'd have taken them to the Citizen's Hospital on the other side of the city, to grey-templed physicians and decades of experience. But then I saw that my newborn twins were trussed up with wires and tubes. A long thin tube went into each tiny mouth conveying oxygen to their lungs. Miniscule intravenous needles were threaded into their veins. Wires linked heartbeats to monitors. Those babies weren't going anywhere. I would have to trust this man.

The Neonatal Intensive Care Unit nurses' photos were tacked to the wall. In several of the snapshots, the nurses were holding a pale-skinned, black-haired baby next to our son's incubator. He was a giant—six or seven pounds at least. Our son weighed less than two pounds.

The nurse in charge of my boy was Ms. Tanaka. She went about her work with the enthusiasm of a kindergarten teacher. She danced with the giant baby from the snapshot to the tune of "Brahm's Lullaby" and took him for "walks." She reached into my son's incubator and made his hand wave as if he were an action figure. "*Genki da yo!*" she said in a baby boy's voice. "Don't worry! I'm fine!"

Sometimes Nurse Tanaka teased Dr. Honda. This seemed bizarre in a country where authority demanded respect. I wondered if they were flirting, even though there is no word for "flirt" in the Japanese language. Most of the NICU staff were young, and I wondered if they had affairs with each other like the nurses and doctors in the American TV show "ER." I wondered if they were married. No rings were allowed in the NICU so it was difficult to tell. No watches, either. Everyone was required to wear a pink smock over their clothes (pink being a colour found to be soothing to babies), and white caps over their hair. The parents wore masks. I had to wash my hands three times before I could touch my babies.

Every three hours, the new mothers gathered in the nursing room to breastfeed our babies. All five or six of us (the number varied) sat on cushioned benches with our pyjamas unbuttoned and our pink or brown nipples bared. There was none of the modesty that

I'd experienced in women's locker rooms in Japan. We compared and admired each others' breasts.

"Mine are so hard," one woman moaned. "Feel them."

At her urging, I pressed the pads of my fingers against her swollen breast and indeed, it was solid.

When the nurse handed over her giant baby boy, she tickled his parted lips with her nipple, but he wouldn't suck. "Don't sleep," she said. "Give me some relief."

I was jealous that she had a baby to suckle, even if he was reluctant. I sat beside her, squeezing colostrum from my own breasts. It slid into the sterilized bottle, thick and yellow, drop by precious drop. My fingers ached. My lily-white breasts were stained with bruises.

I'd heard that thoughts of babies activated the ducts, which made the milk flow faster, so I thought about my son and daughter. My boy had a slender tube through his nose that went directly to his stomach. Every two hours, he was fed two millilitres of my milk. Two cubic centimetres—that's maybe a teardrop or as much dew as falls on one leaf of clover.

That morning, when I'd sat before my daughter's incubator listening to the hum of the respirator, Dr. Honda told me that she could not digest the milk. Although she, too, was fed through a tube that went from her nose to her stomach, the colostrum remained in her stomach, unprocessed. The feeding would be stopped. If she couldn't eat, how would she stay alive?

"I've heard that physical contact can make all the difference with preemies," my college roommate emailed from New York.

I'd heard that too, but I was afraid to touch my babies. I opened the Plexiglas doors to my daughter's incubator and stroked her foot with one finger. She jerked away. Her eyes were still sealed shut. She couldn't look at me. I caressed her arms, ever so lightly, and then her head, and brushed my fingertips over her torso. The monitor alarm went off. I looked up quickly and snatched my hand away when I saw that her heart rate had suddenly dropped from 112 beats per minute to 60.

A nurse came running toward me, rubber soles squeaking on the floor, and then Dr. Honda. "You'd better let her rest awhile," he said. Then he smiled sadly, as if to assure me that it wasn't entirely my fault.

A week after I'd given birth, my mother-in-law arrived in my hospital room with bags of souvenirs. She had spent the previous evening preparing packages of little bean-filled cakes, oranges, and iron-supplemented soft drinks for the visitors sure to stream into my room.

"It's the seventh day," she said knowingly. "And an auspicious day on the calendar."

There was still so much that I didn't know about local tradition, but I was quite sure that no well-wishers would arrive. Later, I would learn that the people in the office where I'd worked had been wondering if my babies were even alive.

It was hard to decide if this was a celebratory occasion or not.

My parents had sent a bouquet of flowers and a card saying "Thank you for our new grandchildren."

My aunt called from Michigan, and her first words were, "I'm so sorry."

My mother-in-law, who was not allowed in the NICU and had not yet seen the babies, knew only that I had provided an heir. She sat by my bed all day and put on her social smile every time the door opened, but my only visitors were the cleaning lady who came to scrub the toilet, the handsome young intern who came to change my IV fluid, the nurse who took my temperature, and a mischievous child who'd barged into the wrong room.

When my husband arrived that evening, my mother-in-law's face was heavy and sad. All of the bags that she had brought remained in a corner of the room.

There was one other woman who expressed milk by hand. Her newborn son (1,318 grams and growing) was in the NICU, too. His incubator was next to my baby girl's.

One day we started talking about mothers-in-law.

I told her how mine sat by my bed all day. "I just want to read my book, but I feel as if I should entertain her. She's always hovering and fussing. If I so much as cough, she jumps up to throw a blanket over me even though I'm sweating. It drives me nuts."

"Mine never visits," the other woman said.

"Why not?"

"Because she blames me for this." And I knew that she was referring to her own defected womb and the tiny boy behind Plexiglas.

On another day, I heard a nurse tell a story of a woman who was divorced for giving birth to a stillborn child. The husband and mother-in-law discussed it while the wife was still convalescing, still grappling with her grief, no doubt. They gave her the news the day after she was released from the hospital. I realized that the woman who annoyed me so much was not so bad after all.

I walked into the NICU in my mask and smock and paper hat, and the young doctor motioned me to his desk.

"Your son in fine," he said. "No problem." And then he took out a photo done by ultrasound, showed me the blue spots that indicated blood in my daughter's lungs. He drew a picture of the heart's chambers and scratched two words above it: "ductus arteriosis." A duct in my daughter's heart had failed to close as it should have after birth. Her body had not adapted to life outside the womb; her lungs didn't understand that they must now fill with oxygen.

The doctor told me that there was medication and, if that didn't work, they could try surgery. He gave me a form to sign my consent.

I sat by her incubator longer than usual that day. "My little sweet pea," I said. "My darling girl." She weighed no more than a small animal—a squirrel, perhaps, or a chipmunk. I could not imagine such a delicate being surviving cuts and sutures.

When I went back to my room, my mother-in-law was plumping pillows and changing the water in the vases of flowers—flowers for "congratulations" and "get well soon."

I tried to smile, but my spirits were flagging. I showed her the form explaining the problem and the procedure for dealing with my baby girl's heart. It was all in Japanese, which I couldn't read. I explained as well as I could that there was a duct that needed to be closed. I tried to be brave and confident because I knew how much my mother-in-law would worry if I wasn't.

The next day when I visited my children, Dr. Honda was listening to opera in his office. I could hear Italians warbling through the partition and tried to identify the music. A tragedy? A comedy? Was this opera one of those stories where the heroine dies consumptive at the end?

The other four babies in the NICU had been released from their Plexiglas prisons. They were given suck at intervals by cheerful moms, taken on promenades by the nurses, bathed in the stainless steel sink. If Dr. Honda was worried, it was because of my children. It was because of the baby girl balanced between heaven and life on earth.

But then the young doctor emerged from his haven and smiled. "Your son," he said, "no problem."

"And my daughter?"

"Getting better."

On the fourth day, the ultrasound revealed that the duct had closed completely. The treatment was a success.

I was exhausted from the midnight, three a.m., and six a.m. milkings, from the heart-pumping drama I'd been forced to endure, and from the bedside hovering of my mother-in-law. When I found her—once again plumping pillows, changing water, rearranging toiletries and so on—I explained in my best Japanese that the duct in my daughter's heart had closed. And then I told her that I wanted to take a nap. She nodded gravely and left me alone in the shuttered room.

I slept. When my mother-in-law returned an hour later, I could see that she had been crying. She told me that she had been wandering the hospital halls worrying about my baby girl.

"The duct closed," I said. "It's a *good* thing."

My daughter was getting better. She was being fed breast milk. She was growing stronger. But then the doctor told me that although the duct in my son's heart had closed on its own, it had now reopened.

"That can happen?" I asked.

"Yes, sometimes. But rarely."

I felt helpless, much as I did when an earthquake rocked our house. Everything was unpredictable, subject to chance.

I was given another form to sign. On this day, I sat next to my son's incubator longer than usual.

On the day that I came home from the hospital, my next-door neighbour was weeding her flower bed. She saw me get out of the car with my little brown suitcase. She looked from my face to my diminished stomach, wiped her hands on her pants, and ambled over.

"Congratulations," she said. "A boy and a girl at once. You're so lucky."

My neighbour had had a baby just this side of forty after years of trying. She was the mother of a five-year-old girl and from what she'd implied, there'd be no more children, no boy. There was an aura of envy around her.

"They're still in the hospital," I said. "They're on life support."

She waved away my concern. "They'll be fine. These days, incubators are just like the mother's womb."

I begged to differ. Inside, the body is warm and dark. The incubator was in brightly lit space. Sometimes the nurses wrapped gauze around my babies' feet and hands because their extremities chilled easily. Inside the body, babies are lulled by the mother's heartbeat and the sound of her voice. The NICU was a cacophony of alarms and beeps and buzzes and infants screaming in pain.

After I left the hospital, everyone I ran into asked, "Why?" "Why did you go into premature labour? Why were your babies born fourteen weeks early?"

My older woman friend thought it was because I let my legs get cold. She'd seen me at a musical in February in a knee-length dress and nothing but nylons when, according to her, I should have been wearing insulated pants.

My boss believed it was because I had walked to work each day—a five minute saunter, if that—carrying a soft-sided briefcase containing notebooks and a magazine or two. He never considered that the cigarette smoke perpetually fogging the office might have had something to do with it. I had a flashback of a cup of coffee downed at my desk in the third month and wondered if that might have been it.

My husband thought it was because I'd gone to an African dance party the week before I started to bleed. I knew when I walked to the bus stop, and later when I boarded the train, that my husband wouldn't approve. But he was in Hokkaido on business, and I would have been alone at home. Better to be among caring friends, I'd thought.

Maybe I shouldn't have moved the furniture when my husband called and said "The new recliner will be delivered in ten minutes. Clear out a space."

But then I thought about my sister-in-law, who'd travelled to Bolivia on business in her seventh month of pregnancy, who'd rested her wine glass on the shelf of her stomach in between sips of Chardonnay, who actually went jogging until a few days before giving birth. Her son, my nephew, was born after two hours of labour. Who was the freak of nature? Me or my sister-in-law? And how can something so ordinary, so natural, go so wrong?

The giant baby was transferred from the NICU to the floor above, to paediatrics. On the day of his departure, I watched his mother dress him in striped blue pyjamas. She packed up his stuffed bear and the mobile that played Brahm's lullaby loud enough for the other babies to hear, and then they were gone.

In a few days the doctor would try to take the tube out of my daughter's lungs.

Without the tube, I could see that my daughter's mouth was shaped like Clara Bow's. It was a beautiful mouth. Until now, she had sucked on the tube for solace, but now she gaped like a fish out of water.

"Her mouth is lonely," the nurse said.

I wished I could slide my pinkie between her lips, but that would be unsanitary.

For the first few hours, she took regular breaths on her own. But in the days that followed, she sometimes forgot to inhale. When she stopped breathing, the monitor beeped. I stepped aside quickly to allow the nurse to reach in and jiggle her. After a moment, her chest rose and fell, and I started breathing again, too. It took a while to get used to it, but I did. Soon, I was the one to reach in and remind her to breathe.

On another day, I was singing to my daughter, making up the words as I went along: "My darling child, my little peanut, my ballerina girl." Suddenly, the doors whooshed open. In came the young doctor, a flock of nurses and a pair of incubators. Another set of twins had been born, alas, too early. I stopped singing and sat frozen like a bird in the bush.

The doctor called out for things, and the nurses handed them over. Each baby was weighed. Within five minutes, both red-skinned newborns had been intubated and set up with IVs. I admired the staff's brisk competence. This must have been what it was like on the day of my babies' birth.

The new twins, two boys, were slightly larger than my son was at birth. My daughter remained the smallest patient in the NICU. I wanted to seek out the parents and tell them that I knew how they felt. "But look!" I'd say. "Our boy was smaller still and now he thrives!" His mouth twitched in a smile. His hand curled around my finger.

The mother was wheeled in on a gurney, up close to the incubators. I watched her reach inside to touch each one and thought, "How lucky! I had to wait till I was able to walk by myself to see my children." But then the heart specialist was called in. He and the other doctors conferred behind screens. They spoke in hushed tones to the twins' parents.

When I visited two days later, one of the new twins was missing. In its place was an incubator covered with vinyl. I knew that it was none of my business, but I gestured and asked, "What happened to the other one?"

The nurse frowned at me. She made a stalling sound—"m-mmm"—and I lowered my eyes.

"Oh," I said. "Pardon me."

In that same week, another baby died, and my daughter's kidneys stopped functioning.

My daughter's face was puffy with water; her diapers remained dry. Two days before, she had been delicate and slender. Now, the nurses joked that she looked like a sumo wrestler.

"We've never seen anything like this before," Dr. Honda told me. "In most cases, kidney failure occurs immediately after birth, not two months later."

"What's causing it?" I asked.

He answered with the most chilling words yet: "We don't know."

This was a country where doctors pretended to be gods, a condition that made his frankness all the more alarming. For once in my life, I would have preferred a lie, some fake confidence.

When milk time came around, my daughter got nothing. She was being fed intravenously until her condition improved.

The doctor told us that our son was almost ready to go home. I had nearly forgotten that these days would end, that my husband and I were the true guardians of the baby boy and girl in the incubators. The thought of taking care of them by ourselves—the responsibility—terrified me.

I was sitting, watching my daughter's miniature chest rise and fall, when I saw something black out of the corner of my eye. It was a fly. I thought, at first, that it was in the incubator with my baby, but then I noticed that it was crawling up the blinds.

"Hey!" I called out, in a panic. "There's a fly in here!" Flies carried germs. Flies caused African sleeping sickness, which was unlikely here in rural Japan, but who knew what other vector-borne diseases there were that could kill my children.

One of the nurses, who was always impeccably made up, strolled over. "Where?" she asked. Her voice was calm.

I pointed to the winged vermin now exploring the top of my daughter's incubator.

The nurse took a rolled up notebook and swatted. The fly was dead. I breathed a sigh of relief.

"How'd it get in here?" I asked. The windows were sealed.

"It must have followed one of you mothers in here," she said. "Maybe it liked the smell of your milk."

A couple of days later, when I went to another part of the hospital for insurance purposes, I saw a kitten in the corridor. A kitten: fleas, mites, toxoplasmosis. "Nurse," I called out to a young woman in starched white. "There's a cat in here!"

The nurse looked in the direction I'd indicated. "So there is," she said with a smile. "How cute!" And then, believe it or not, she walked away, off to the ladies' room.

I wondered if I was being paranoid. I wondered if I would be able to protect my son—and later my daughter—from all the black flies and kittens and other dangers in the world.

My son began breathing room air, unassisted. He was taken out of the incubator and installed in a Plexiglas bed. He started drinking breast milk from a bottle and then, little by little, from my breast. He cried loudly whenever he was hungry, and I worried that he might be disturbing the other babies who were weaker and sicker.

Dr. Honda told us that when our baby boy reached 2,500 grams, he could go home. He now tipped the scale at 2,300.

We hadn't finished preparing the nursery yet, but this news brought a bloom to my cheeks. It had been almost three months since he'd departed my body, and I longed to have him close again.

Dr. Honda asked if we'd like to schedule our son's release for an auspicious day on the Japanese calendar. I was not superstitious like my mother-in-law, but I knew that she would be horrified if our son left the NICU on an unlucky day. I was not superstitious, but I was willing to take all the help I could get.

The medicine that the doctors prescribed for our daughter had worked. Her kidneys were functioning properly once again and her second chin had melted. Her milk intake had increased. She was getting better, but I took nothing for granted. There had been too many surprises along the way. Every day my husband chanted Buddhist sutras, and I prayed to God while on my knees.

A few weeks later, my daughter began to acquire the suggestion of meat around her thighs. At last, she developed a labia and grew eyelashes.

By the time that our son was ready to check out of the hospital, our tiny baby girl was out of the incubator as well, engulfed in a gauze kimono and swaddled in a white bath towel.

I dressed my son in baby clothes for the first time. The little sailor outfit was intended for a preemie, but it was roomy on my boy.

My husband and I gave the NICU staff a box of cream puffs and a case of soft drinks as an infinitesimal token of our appreciation. Insurance had pretty much picked up the tab for our children's care, but we wanted to pay back something.

Everyone gathered round as we prepared to take our boy out. I couldn't speak because my throat was jammed shut by emotion. Instead, I bowed and let the doctors and nurses see the tears in my eyes.

I said "good-bye for today" to my daughter and tucked my son into a wicker basket with a comforter printed with a teddy bear motif. I carried him out the whooshing door. When I stepped onto the elevator with my baby boy in a basket, it felt as if I were doing something illegal.

I could now hold, feed, and bathe my son whenever I wanted to. The nurses no longer had any say. Dr. Honda's work was done. Now it was up to us to keep him alive. It was late summer, and the sun shone on my child for the first time.

My daughter was released from the hospital a month later around the time when the nights began to cool, and the leaves began to crisp. We would later find out that, due to her premature birth, she was deaf and had cerebral palsy. During the first three years of her life, she would be admitted to the hospital ten times for various respiratory ailments. Now both twins are healthy and happy teenagers. We are indeed lucky.

Names have been changed to protect the identities of the individuals mentioned in this essay.

4.
A Triography of Polymaternity

Becoming Mamas to Triplets

ABIGAIL L. PALKO

A S AMERICAN MOTHERING PRACTICES in the twenty-first century evolve to reflect social changes—including growing visibility of lesbian-headed families, blended families, and families formed through assisted reproductive technologies—one crucial component to new understandings of maternal identities must be individual women's specific stories of their lived realities. In her study of queer mothering practices, Shelley M. Park argues that the "polymaternal" family "is a queer family structure that requires the queering of intimacy in triangulated—or even more complex—relations of mothers and child(ren)" (1). Accordingly, this essay centres on a newly married lesbian couple's experience of becoming mothers to triplets, conceived via assisted reproductive technology (ART), to focus on the intersections of the experiences of lesbian mothering and of mothering multiples. I draw on Park's articulation of "monomaternalism" and follow her lead in queering mothering practices.

By its very nature as polymaternal, lesbian mothering invites the question, "who is the 'real' mother?" This question, as Park notes, is threatening: "what is at stake in our claims about 'real' mothers is the notion that children must have *one and only one* mother. Heteronormative power cannot countenance polymaternal families and practices of child rearing" (3). In the ethnographic triography that follows, I demonstrate how polymaternal families also have the power to disrupt notions of what maternal practice "looks like"; this disruption is potentially intensified in families of multiples.

This essay takes the form of a triography[1], an ethnography in triplicate. I use the term "triography" to capture the tripartite creation of knowledge and understanding that my methodology entails: I undertook an extended in-person interview with the couple, Meg and Julia; for this initial interview, although I had questions prepared[2], my intention was to prompt the interviewees to speak freely and broadly about their maternal experiences raising their four sons (the older boy, whom I refer to as FB, or firstborn, was born to Meg and her previous partner). I then shaped their responses into a narrative, intercut with insights from the published scholarly literature on lesbian mothers.[3] In the writing process, I posed additional questions via email, which we discussed over the phone. Finally, when the essay draft was complete, I sent it to Meg and Julia to ensure that it reflected their perception of their maternal identities. My goal throughout the process has been to honour their knowledge as equally important (if not more so) as the scholarship that I bring to the project, amplifying their voices and highlighting their lived experiences.

In a culture (the United States) that for decades has privileged an isolated form of mothering in which a single woman takes on exclusive mothering responsibilities, how do two women negotiate the development of maternal identities? And how is this process complicated by the presence of multiple infants in twin or triplet births? This latter question is particularly salient given the increase in planned lesbian-headed families through ART, which itself carries a greater than average chance of multiple births. A number of studies discuss important issues that lesbian mothers face but do not consider the impact of multiparous births.[4] Furthermore, the existing research is concerned with the impact of mothers' sexual orientation on their children (Golombok and Badger); few studies consider how the co-mother feels about the experience, and this present study seeks to suggest ways to fill this gap. As my interest in this project is the rhetorical construction of identity, it seems crucial that the mothers' voices themselves take priority in the account. As an ethnography of one particular couple, this account should not be considered a universal standard. But in telling their story, Meg and Julia suggest fruitful avenues for further research, particularly at the intersection of the experiences of lesbian mothering and mothering multiples. I am not alone in observing that feminist studies of mothering practices frequently elide the lesbian mother in their heteronormativity (Park); this elision is particularly pronounced in studies of mothers of multiples. As Laura Mamo reminds us, lesbian mothering is not a new practice. The newness factor lies in the technology that has offered a solution to a biological need (for sperm) that has not actually precluded lesbian mothering in the past. This technological development has, however, produced new meanings, as donor insemination has been biomedicalized (Mamo 195), leading to a greatly increased potential for multiples.

PREGNANT WITH TRIPLETS[5]

When Meg and Julia decided to add to their family, the decision to use the leftover sperm from when Meg had conceived her first son (with her previous partner, who has visitation rights) was simple: this way, although the family would not all be biologically related, the children would share the same genetic father.[6] So they embarked on several rounds of intrauterine insemination (IUI), with Meg as the selected biological mother. The midwife asked if Julia would be nursing, too, and, more significantly, Meg herself offered to gestate the pregnancy using Julia's eggs. But for Julia, pregnancy and biological motherhood were "never in the cards." The women thus selected a more "traditional" form of donor-inseminated pregnancy. Spanish doctors have developed the Reception of Oocytes from Partner (ROPA) technique, or Partner Assisted Reproduction, whereby both partners in a lesbian relationship can be biological mothers: one woman serves as the gestating mother and the other one donates the eggs. S. Marina and colleagues present this as a way for lesbians to share not only their lives and sexuality but also biological maternity (940). Their description of the technique's benefits, however, prioritizes biological maternity in an essentialist way that does not resonate with Julia. Marina et. al. write, "Both of the women in lesbian couples who request the ROPA technique wish to share in the maternity experience, instead of having one partner be a mere spectator, as happens with DI [donor insemination]" (940). Neither Meg nor Julia would characterize Julia as a "mere spectator": Meg talks lovingly of the ways that Julia was involved in the pregnancy, including reading all of the books. For Julia, the decision was clear and easy; the fact that, because the women are legally married in their home state, they were listed as the triplets' two parents on their birth certificates at birth surely removed any legal incentive there might otherwise have been for Julia to take on a biological role. As their example demonstrates, "sharing" the pregnancy is not a necessary precursor to ensuring that the non-gestating partner is not a "mere spectator," particularly for couples who do not ascribe to monomaternalism.

Monomaternalism, as Park defines it, refers to the "ideological assumption that a child can have only one real mother" (3); this stems from both social norms and (presumed) biological imperatives. She further posits that "Assertions about who is or is not a 'real' mother often carry normative weight similarly intended to discipline those who deviate from norms of femininity" (3-4). There is also an important racial-cultural component to monomaternalism, as Park lays it out: not all cultures in the United States subscribe to this ideology, of course. In the African American community, for example, women have long relied on *Othermothers* to share maternal responsibilities, as Patricia Hill Collins has demonstrated. Park further argues,

> Monomaternalism, as an ideological doctrine, resides at the intersection of patriarchy (with its insistence that women bear responsibility for biological and social reproduction), heteronormativity (with its insistence that a woman must pair with a man, rather than with other women, in order to raise children successfully), capitalism (in its conception of children as private property), and Eurocentrism (in its erasure of polymaternalism in other cultures and historical periods). (7)

Cultural discussions of mothering practices often lead to claims about what constitutes a "real mother"; in turn, such constructions often depend on participation in specific biological processes (Park 4). For lesbian co-mothers, however, active participation in these processes can only occur via technological interventions. For Meg and Julia, then, once they decided that Meg would carry their pregnancy, Julia's few options for biological involvement were to serve as egg donor, a highly invasive procedure, or to stimulate lactation to nurse, another hormonally invasive procedure. For women unwilling or unable to undergo these bodily invasions, motherhood must be conceived of through alternate routes. Park compares this process to the one faced by stepmothers: "Lesbian co-mothers often encounter a similar phenomenon, wherein the status of their relationship to the child borne of their partner is queried and they find themselves named (sometimes by their own partners or ex-partners) as something other than mother" (5). Here, Sara Ruddick's work on maternal thinking is particularly instructive.

In her groundbreaking *Maternal Thinking*, Ruddick identifies three goals of maternal practice: protection, nurturance, and training; these goals are designed to meet the social demands of preservation, growth, and acceptability (23). Maternal thinking, she argues, not only creates strategies to achieve these ends, but in the process also creates maternal identity. For Ruddick, maternal identity is not rooted in the biological; in fact, she claims, "In any culture, maternal commitment is far more voluntary than people like to believe" (22). A mother, she posits, is "a person who takes on responsibility for children's lives and for whom providing child care is a significant part of her or his working life" (40). She is careful (and adamant!) to confirm that her gender expansiveness is deliberate: for Ruddick, the mother is the person, female or male, who actively, purposefully chooses to mother. She defines mothering by the practices involved rather than the biological processes. And because mothering is a deliberate choice, she argues that all mothers are adoptive, even if they have gestated and given birth to their children (51). This perspective opens the possibility that multiple people can assume maternal responsibility for a child, as in the case of lesbian co-mothers. Beyond the legal aspect, Julia was clear that for her, motherhood was not something she anticipated undertaking:

> For me, I internalized the media telling you [that] you can't. I didn't think in my lifetime that I could. Then I really took a step back and thought, I looked at the people I worked

with. I saw how it is this awesome responsibility and how many people didn't take it seriously—if these people can do it, I can do it, why did I think I didn't have the skills? I realized it was more of the media and society dictating and suppressing ideas because I didn't think I could have it.

Julia's reflections demonstrate maternal thinking in progress: after considering and rejecting normative notions of appropriate maternal identity, Julia chose to take responsibility for their future child(ren), in effect adopting them (à la Ruddick) prior to conception. For Julia, the non-biological mother, her maternal identity seems to have been firmly established by her acceptance of Ruddick's tasks and goals.

Since being married in 2012, the question of whether or not to have more children has been a negotiation in Meg and Julia's relationship. Meg always wanted one more child so that FB could have a sibling. But she wanted to marry Julia more than she wanted to have more children, so they got engaged with the idea that they would not be having more kids. FB was a year old when they met, and Meg got rid of all of his baby things. Ultimately, though, Julia changed her mind. She explained, "I changed my mind because we had told two people that we were contemplating having kids and then they both died the same day." In this loss, they saw a sign that they should welcome another child into their lives. But in Julia's explanation, I also heard a sense that she had become a maternal figure in FB's life and this allowed her to consider the possibility. Meg sees this as well; after our last conversation, she emailed me to add, "One more thing ... I never would've pushed Julia to have more children; but after seeing her with FB and how terrific she was and how well we complemented each other as parents, I was hopeful that she would change her mind on her own." When I asked Julia what FB calls her, she shared that at first she was just "Jules" but that she became "Mama Jules" because she had earned the right to be a variation of "mom." With the triplets, who are not speaking yet, they are still working out who will have what name, although Meg is adamant that she hates mommy, feeling that then "mother" ceases to be an adult identity. For now, she refers to herself as Mama.

The question of names cuts to the heart of the identity issue that this essay explores. For Meg, her maternal identity is easy, firm. Although both women are well-educated with professional careers, Meg is staying at home for now. In the beginning, the sheer logistics of daycare for triplets, with the attendant costs, was further complicated by health issues that two of the boys and Meg all had following the pregnancy. When I asked them to describe their roles, Meg explained, "At the moment I'm the stay-at-home mom, also known by my wife as 'Dairy Queen.' It's very much the 'mother-role' with the exception that I'm in charge of all the bills. I'm the CEO of the house. I'm not a cleaner. She's OCD. I always feel guilty for having any mess." Her job is currently being held for her, and while she regrets that they cannot make the decision freely, economic considerations will most likely be the deciding factor in the decision about when she returns.

Because Julia is the co-mother, her role is not so easily inscribed. The fact that Meg had FB before she met Julia further complicates Julia's maternity in some ways: with FB, she eased into a maternal role, and with the triplets, she assumed it prior to efforts to conceive them. When I asked Julia to describe her role, I heard in her answer some of the uncertainties that she also expressed elsewhere. She is aware that she has very much taken on the male-father role: "I'm the breadwinner, I feel that responsibility. I like my job, I need it. I'm responsible for four children. When I come home, I play with the kids. Doesn't get more ... even yard work. I do it. I like it. I hate the kitchen. If you look at the old traditional. It's just that very traditional. Which is fine with me." We talked about whether she assumed the traditionally "masculine" role because she never thought that she would become a mother or because that was the only reasonable course of action once they were faced with triplets. Julia's answer points to a generous way out of the interminable "Mommy Wars" that have shaped contemporary American mothering practices:

I think it's my personality. Even now if someone said you have the choice between staying home with them or going to work, I know I would work. She enjoys it and is excellent. I think people should gravitate toward what they feel more comfortable with. I certainly love them to death. But someone has to make the money. Even if my salary wasn't as high, I would still see myself going to work and Meg staying home with them. Meg works; she has the hardest job here. I get a break. I have the drive to and from work without people crying, grabbing me. It's a role I feel comfortable with. It seems instinctual. I never second-guessed it. It was comfortable for us.

The question of how the co-mother develops her maternal identity seems to be one of the greatest benefits to having triplets: the sheer logistics of caring for three newborns leaves no room for angst about division of labour in the way that Meg and Julia tell the story, and each is free (in Julia's words) to "gravitate toward" her strengths.

Because she is not the biological mother, Julia has some flexibility in negotiating her maternal identity, but with flexibility comes other issues, however. She is clear that the role of stay-at-home mother is not the right role for her: "If I had to stay home with them ... I know my limitations. I'd rather work fourteen hours [a day]," she readily admits. The day-to-day care of the triplets (as infants) is, she said, "Way harder than any career I could imagine—and I like work and I like hard work." She expressed clear empathy for Meg's daily reality: "I feel badly for Meg—every morning this is all day with three of them. They are not napping yet." At the same time, Julia faces other challenges that Meg does not. Meg shared: "It was particularly difficult for her during the pregnancy and the immediate birth because she was not out at work. The stress was just stress. That was tougher than it needed to be—because of that situation." For a variety of complicated reasons, Julia was not able to use *Family and Medical Leave Act* (FMLA) time off after the triplets' birth; she was only able to get a little time to see Meg (who had medical complications from the pregnancy) and even that required delicate negotiation. Julia also has to negotiate public questions about her maternal status; Meg observed, "I think it's hysterical when Julia is out with the triplets and she's pushing the stroller and people are like, aw triplets. You look great for having triplets." Comments about her maternal status have not yet been accompanied by judgements about her parenting skills. Thus, although studies have indicated that "lesbian social mothers feel the need to justify the quality of their parenthood" (Bos, van Balen, and van den Boom 761), Julia did not express any such concern, which might be another side benefit to having triplets: there is no time to worry about whether she is mothering "properly"—she has to just mother.

Meg is aware of Julia's recognition of the intensity of the labour that she puts in as the stay-at-home mother in the family. Having co-mothered with her ex-partner, she has a base of comparison. Meg articulated clear differences in the two experiences, some of which are based on personality differences: "[the experiences are] vastly different. Julia has more of an appreciation for the parenting aspect. My ex was also jealous that I wasn't working. She was actually visibly irritable about wanting to spend money like it was on trees instead of acknowledging that we needed money for diapers. Julia calls it our money. With my ex, it was her money." But other differences between the two experiences—important differences, all three of us would argue—are the result of having triplets: "Because there are three, there's no way for me to physically take care of all three and there's much more involvement with Julia. That started in the beginning when the oldest triplet refused to nurse. She gave him pumped breast milk. We established a better routine in the beginning to do better parenting." I asked whether this was because it was Meg's second time or because they had triplets. She laughed and said "Yes," before elaborating, "There is some difference for the fact there are three, but I think the other difference is how she came to want to have children and she was determined not to mess this up." From Meg's perspective, Julia committed to a maternal identity prior to the triplets' birth, and as a result, she has been a full partner from the very beginning.

From observations she makes among her fellow participants in a local Facebook group for mothers of multiples, Meg sees a difference between Julia's co-parenting style and that of the fathers discussed in the group[7]:

> One of the best things I can do is leave her alone with them for a few hours to remind her [how hard it is]. It's fascinat-

ing because I'm not sure it's how men would approach it. Some men on the Facebook group don't necessarily get it. At no point has Julia given me a "honey-do" list—there isn't a stress put on that. There are days that things go crazy—things are not so neat.

In Meg's perception (and Julia's comments confirm this), Julia comprehends the work involved just in caring for the three boys with a depth of understanding that fathers often do not have.

In our extended interview, Meg and Julia did not discuss the fact that their children do not have a social father. Early research on lesbian co-mothers focused on the impact on children that the absence of a male parental figure caused. In a 1997 study, A. Brewaeys et. al. argue that the absence of a biologically male father does not negatively impact children raised in lesbian families. The study, although outdated, usefully confirms assertions that the presence of two mothers does not harm children through its delineation of the impact of the roles played by social mothers: "Both women in the lesbian mother family were actively engaged in child care and a strong mutual attachment had developed between social mother and child" (1356). The researchers' framework presumes a conservative vision of the father's role—one analogous to that articulated by Sara Ruddick as the "capital-F" father (42-43)— which they describe as "a symbol of authority responsible for the introduction of prohibitions and limitations" (1349). Such a view of the paternal role suggests that children raised without father figures are at a significant disadvantage, an argument that critics of same-sex families routinely make. Brewaeys et. al. find, however, that the social mothers (as they term co-mothers) in their study were "significantly more involved" in both practical child-care activities and disciplinary activities than were the fathers in either heterosexual control groups (1354). They note measurable differences between social mothers and fathers:

However, one striking difference was found between lesbian and heterosexual families: social mothers showed greater interaction with their children than did fathers. Interestingly, the quality of parent-child interaction did not differ significantly between the two mothers in lesbian families, but in both heterosexual groups mothers interacted more with their children than did fathers. (1356)

Brewaeys et al. argue that the social mother is by her nature as a female more invested in her children's welfare than the father in his: "The fact that the other parent is also a woman makes her role in the lesbian family essentially different from that of the father in a heterosexual family in that her investment in the child is stronger" (1356); the difference in involvement in their children stems, they argue, from the parent's gender identity, not his or her sexual orientation. Brewaeys et. al. argue, "The different position of the social mother in lesbian families compared with that of fathers in heterosexual families is confirmed by the division of professional and childcare activities between the two parents" (1356). This study, however, again assumes a singleton child. The case of Meg and Julia, however, suggests that an important factor in how couples undertake the division of labour is determined by the number of children involved as well as, perhaps, the mothers' earlier socialization toward maternal impulses. Julia has developed her own maternal identity: she provides breadwinning work, support for Meg in the daily caretaking work, and then caretaking of her own when she is home from work.

BECOMING THE CO-MOTHER

In a study of twenty-four (largely) middle-to-upper-class co-mothers (defined as "women who self-identified as lesbian non-biological mothers in a committed relationship" [53]) in the Pacific Northwest, Danuta M. Wojnar and Amy Katzenmeyer conducted descriptive phenomenological inquiries to explore the conception, pregnancy, and postpartum experiences of non-biological mothers. They found that "an overarching sense of 'feeling different' permeated the experiences of pre-pregnancy through new motherhood" for the women with whom they spoke (53). They contend that transitioning into motherhood emphasized non-biological mothers' otherness in terms of mainstream society; this difference was exacerbated by biological and legal issues: "they had a desire to parent but they were unable to contribute biologically and were not protected legally until the adoption process was complete" (58). In Meg and Julia's case, Julia did not have to legally adopt the triplets but rather was named on their birth certificates from the outset. She did not express the angst that Wojnar and Katzenmeyer discuss, emphasizing the power of legal uncertainty to unsettle maternal identity. Furthermore, Wojnar and Katzenmeyer suggest that non-biological lesbian mothers face a "complex" path to motherhood, a process complicated not only by the legal and biological factors but also by a dearth of role models and an attendant sense of isolation and invisibility (58). The result, they argue, is that the non-biological mother has to create a unique maternal role within society and her family in the face of a "pervasive feeling of otherness and the complexity of [their] emotions surrounding parenthood, in particular during the postpartum period" (59).

In their study, Wojnar and Katzenmeyer assert an insecurity on the part of the co-mothers that I did not see in speaking with Meg and Julia. Wojnar and Katzenmeyer found that the women in their study worried about becoming attached to their children and found the bonding process difficult because of a lack of biological connection (56). Attachment, for the lesbian co-mothers, occurred in a manner analogous to paternal experiences: "attachment happened gradually through typical child care, such as rocking the infant and changing diapers" (56). And even once the lesbian co-mothers had bonded with their children, they still expressed a sense of distance: "there was still a pervasive feeling that the biological mother had a connection with the child that the non-biological mother could never attain" (56). Wojnar and Katzenmeyer thus highlight difficulties in bonding that the co-mother might potentially face if motherhood is considered through an essentialized biological lens. Given the rise of planned lesbian-headed families, though, one should ask if these norms will continue to hold true. Mamo argues that "the present is productive of new reproductive subjectivities and material practices" (226). Developments of assisted reproductive technologies of the past two decades have in turn contributed to the evolution of lesbian reproduction, such that today it "tends to be a highly biomedicalized process" (226), as it was for Meg and Julia.

Mamo's insightful analysis of the use of donor matching in lesbian reproduction highlights the kinship work that this decision undertakes. Meg and Julia's description of their choice of donor for the triplets illustrates the concept of "affinity ties," which Mamo defines as the "deliberate construction of relatedness enabled through assemblages of meanings of blood, genes, and social and cultural connection" (231). Thus, Mamo finds that "These practices are pragmatic negotiations in which lesbians ask two questions: will the child be accepted as mine? And will the child be similar enough to me and my family to be accepted as ours?" (190-1). The concept of "affinity ties," as Mamo further develops it, does not depend on physical appearance. Equally important is the "imagined future connection forged through shared ancestry, hobbies, and other more cultural attributes" (205). "Affinity ties," she argues, "function as a kinship device in contexts of uncertain legal rights and social legitimacy" (205). As the years since the publication of Mamo's text have brought both growing social acceptance of same-sex parents and new legal protections to lesbian co-mothers (including the 2015 United States Supreme Court ruling legalizing same-sex marriage, announced while this essay was in the final stages of preparation), such a construction is seemingly becoming less necessary from a legal standpoint. Meg is clear that she wanted FB to have a full sibling, and Julia agreed; in their case, affinity ties seem to be activated for sibling bonding purposes.

CONCLUSION

Having triplets has both blessed and challenged Meg and Julia. At the time of our initial interview, they were still in the postpartum throes of adapting to life with newborns. When I asked about the impact on their relationship, they spoke wistfully of the couple time they had temporarily lost: "Lying in bed, we miss each other. We don't have any meaningful conversation about us. One day." In a follow-up conversation, just before the triplets' first birthday, Julia reported that they were sleeping through the night and just starting to walk (but not super mobile yet). At this moment in time, she said, "I can right now feel like I can use that word [easier]. The first months, I would never ever want to relive again. Now, I feel like, if there is such a thing as easy with triplets [she laughed], it's easier than the early months." Julia was aware that this balance is precarious and can change at any moment. There is still always work to be done, though, which comes at the expense of spending quiet time together. Getting time out without the children is also a challenge; they only have one friend who can handle staying alone with the triplets, so going out typically requires lining up two babysitters.

But they also expressed a new compassion for other people facing fertility challenges. Julia told me, "You can read [people's faces] now—people look sad"; they have developed an intuition about how people react to their triplets, a sense of who is struggling to form a family. When I asked what the biggest challenge(s) are that they face, they thought immediately of the logistical issues that mothering multiples pose: as Julia said, "there are two of us and three of them, and the guilt that ensues" from being unable to immediately respond at times. They reflected on a deeper sense of guilt as well. Meg shared, "It's obviously a blessing. I think of the people who can't have children, and I wonder why we have three and some can't have any. I have to believe something is working up there." But they also described joyful moments as the boys develop. After initial health scares, they are now all at home, and Meg and Julia can watch their older son care for and be loving towards the triplets, noting that "He clearly models how we care for them." Now that the triplets are old enough to know each other and look for each other, Meg and Julia have identified another benefit to having triplets; as they described the triplets interacting, I caught a note of hope that the boys will become companions for each other as they get older, which in turn would ease some of the guilt Julia mentioned and the pressure on their relationship.

Park argues that:

> To queer our notions of mothering, however, we cannot attend merely to ways in which the presence of multiple mothers affects the child. A purely child-centered approach to mothering too easily recuperates polymaternalism into

99

heteronormative family structures and affective relations wherein the mother-child dyad remains primary and becomes the site of contestation between mothers. A queer account of mothering needs to explore the third arm of the mother-mother-child triangle, namely the affective relationship between the mothers themselves. (11)

Thoughtful consideration of the impact of mothering multiples on lesbian mothering practices can help to queer our understanding of mothering in the ways that Park advocates. The mere presence of multiples also shatters the mother-child dyad; lesbian co-mothers and a multiparous pregnancy create a web of relationships that makes room for a much wider variety of maternal identities, particularly when the goals of maternal thinking laid out by Ruddick are accounted for. For starters, preservation takes on new salience and urgency, ironically leaving less time for thoughtful, considered construction of maternal identities. Instead, if Meg and Julia are at all representative, lesbian co-mothers of multiples more easily assume maternal identities because there is an increased need and demand for maternal action. On a related note, Park forces us to consider the consequences of broadening our concept of maternal love to incorporate the mothers' bond, asking, "What would happen if maternal love was configured not only (or even primarily) as a putatively unconditional bond between a woman and her offspring, but also as an affectionate—and perhaps even erotic—relationship between mothers?" (12).

Concluding her final email to me Meg wrote, "We call ourselves the best teammates ever now. We have sincerely become terrific teammates in this whole process. This sets the stage for some solid consistency for our children"; this bonding has come specifically through their co-mothering relationship. As Meg and Julia's story so poignantly illustrates, maternal identity formation among lesbian co-mothers can be figured by a multitude of moments in which each woman embraces maternal responsibilities.

This study was approved by the Institutional Review Board at my home institution.

NOTES

[1]To the best of my knowledge, David Leddick coined the word "triography" for the subtitle of *Intimate Companions*, a biography of the photographer George Platt Lynes, the painter Paul Cadmus, and the critic Lincoln Kirstein. His intended meaning differs from mine, though, in that he employs the prefix "tri" to signify three subjects, as opposed to my indication of three creators of knowledge.

[2]These questions were:

Describe your parental role.

Describe your decision to become parents via ART.

What will the children call you (when they start speaking)?

How did you decide on this name?

When did you find out that you were expecting triplets?

What benefits to triplets have you experienced? What challenges?

Have you noticed changes to your relationship with your wife? How would you describe these changes?

[3]I would like to thank Meg and Julia, who so generously and graciously opened their home and family to me.

[4]In fact, I was quite surprised at the current paucity of research on lesbian mothers of multiples.

[5]When asked if they expected to have triplets, Meg and Julia told the story in an amused, the joke's on us manner. The triplets weren't conceived in initial rounds of IUI, and they were running low on sperm. While they could have purchased more, they realized that they were running out of time to have a full biological sibling for their older child. They switched to in vitro fertilization (IVF); two embryos, an eight cell one and a fifteen cell one, were put in, with the hope that one would implant. And then the joke began: both implanted, and an early ultrasound showed twins. The following week, Meg went alone to a doctor's appointment; Julia didn't hear from Meg and began to worry. Meg arrived home and Julia questioned if both were okay. Meg simply held up three fingers. And herein lies the heart of the joke: neither had considered the possibility that they would have multiples, despite the fact that they are both twins. (Meg is an identical twin; Julia is a fraternal twin.) Definitely, Julia had no thought

that two eggs would result in three children.

[6]When Meg first selected the sperm, she purposefully chose a donor open to being contacted when the child turns eighteen so that he not be denied access to his full genetic history. His paternal genetic history is, as she framed it, "a major part of his medical history and I thought it would be unfair for him not to have his full medical history," since her own mother had died when she was twenty-five. In this decision, Meg revealed a bifurcated understanding of family formation that clearly delineates between parental status and genetic inheritance.

[7]Although exploring this observation in further depth is well beyond the scope of this essay, there are a number of elements in it that would make fruitful grounds for further study, most notably: is there a gendered difference in the co-parents' approach and/or in the biological mothers' descriptions of their involvement?

WORKS CITED

Bos, Henry M. W., Fran van Balen, and Dymphna C. van den Boom. "Experience of Parenthood, Couple Relationship, Social Support, and Child-rearing Goals in Planned Lesbian Mother Families." *Journal of Child Psychology and Psychiatry* 45.4 (2004): 755-64. Web. 3 September 2014.

Brewaeys, A., I. Ponjaert, E. V. Van Hall, and S. Golombok. "Donor Insemination: Child Development and Family Functioning in Lesbian Mother Families." *Human Reproduction* 12.6 (1997): 1349-59. Web. 3 September 2014.

Collins, Patricia Hill. *Black Feminist Thought: Knowledge, Consciousness, and the Politics of Empowerment.* 2nd ed. New York: Routledge, 2000. Print.

Golombok, Susan and Shirlene Badger. "Children Raised in Mother-headed Families from Infancy: a Follow-up of Children of Lesbian and Single Heterosexual Mothers, at Early Adulthood." *Human Reproduction* 25.1 (2010): 150-7. Web. 3 September 2014.

Mamo, Laura. *Queering Reproduction: Achieving Pregnancy in the Age of Technoscience.* Durham: Duke University Press, 2007. Print.

Marina, S., D. Marina, F. Marina, N. Fosas, N. Galiana, and I. Jove. "Sharing Motherhood: Biological Lesbian Co-mothers, a New IVF Indication." *Human Reproduction* 25.4 (2010): 938-41. Web. 3 September 2014.

Park, Shelley M. *Mothering Queerly, Queering Motherhood: Resisting Monomaternalism in Adoptive, Lesbian, Blended, and Polygamous Families.* Albany: Suny Press, 2013. Print.

Pawelski, James G. et. al. "The Effects of Marriage, Civil Union, and Domestic Partnership Laws on the Health and Well-being of Children." *Pediatrics* 118.1 (July 2006): 349-64. Web. 3 September 2014.

Ruddick, Sara. *Maternal Thinking: Toward a Politics of Peace.* 1989. Boston: Beacon Press, 1995. Print.

Wojnar, Danuta M. and Amy Katzenmeyer. "Experiences of Preconception, Pregnancy, and New Motherhood for Lesbian Nonbiological Mothers." *Journal of Obstetric, Gynecologic, & Neonatal Nursing* 43.1 (January/February 2014): 50–60. Web. 3 November 2014.

5.
Notes from the Night Owl Feed

KIRSTEN EVE BEACHY

SECOND BREAKFAST
Irene: Left + two oz bottle
Sallie: Right 20 diligent minutes
Pump: skipped

It's breakfast again. I get organized in the nursing rocker that Aunt Loretta brought us. It has no arms, which makes it easy to position the tandem nursing pillow and adjust the strap around my ever-evolving waist. The rocking armchair from Aunt Jewel, just across the living room, is better for actually rocking Irene when she screams all evening.

I tuck a folded flannel blanket into Sallie's side of the pillow to catch the drips and ready the nipple shield for Irene. "Baby me!" I order Jason, and he scoops his oldest daughter out of the cradle where she has been fussing and hands her to me. I tuck Irene under my arm, and she burrows toward my nipple. I have only seconds to help her get a good latch before her angry headshaking starts and she knocks off the shield. This time, we're lucky. She clamps on, and my milk flows quickly. I won't have to syringe milk under the shield to keep her interest.

Jason brings Sallie, and I add another shield and nudge her into place, hoping not to dislodge Irene. With her low muscle tone, she needs back support and a finger under her chin to reinforce her latch. She's wide awake for once, and chomps away with more interest than expertise. Some of the milk is going down her throat, I think.

104

Jason waits with a back-up bottle in the battered recliner where I have been sleeping. It hurts to lie down post-Caesarean. When Aunt Mim comes to help, she will buy us yet another rocking chair, a big leather recliner, and we will squeeze it into this little room alongside the cradle, the bassinet, the woodstove, the couch, the armchair, and the two other rockers.

LUNCH
Irene: Right +1
Sallie: +2 oz
Pump: 2.5

Sallie is working hard at her bottle, trying to hold it all together—the suck, the swallow. Milk drips out around her tongue. She'll manage a couple of ounces. In the bassinet beside me, Irene awakens and stretches, a mighty stretch with one arm back and the other forward, like a warrior, an archer. In a moment, she will start to roar. She is fierce and wonderful. My gaze falls back to Sallie's small face, her limp arms, her elfin ear. She is soft and vulnerable.

My lion. My lamb.

I bought the palm-sized wire-bound notebook weeks before their birth to record my improvised notes on breastfeeding times, pumping, and supplemental bottle feeds. I printed out charts to hang above the changing table where we could keep a tally of diaper changes and drew a diagram of where all the baby clothes belonged. There's even a little note clarifying which diaper balm is compatible with our cloth diapers. On the refrigerator are lists for household helpers. My calendar has different aunts, grandmothers, sisters, and cousins scheduled to stay with us for a full three months. Our church family signed up to bring us meals three times a week for three months. I stocked up on toothpaste and detergent to last for months. You might say I was prepared.

I was not prepared for Sallie's diagnosis.

Neither was the girls' doctor in the hospital, a kindly country doctor we had chosen because we didn't want to drive twenty minutes into town for all their appointments. He didn't disclose his suspicions about Down syndrome until two days after they were born, not until Jason urged him to explain Sallie's low muscle tone.

At the girls' first check-up, the doctor's partner cheerfully presented the possibility that Sallie might not have Down syndrome. Sure, her eyes and face had the classic shape, but he thought she looked a lot like Jason. It took us a month to find a competent pediatrician and have her diagnosis confirmed via genetic testing, a simple blood test we could have had at the hospital, had we known, had anyone offered.

THE FEED OF MILK AND COOKIES
Irene: Left — nursing all the time! So much spit up.
Sallie: Right +3 oz
Pump: 4 oz

It is bad form to get crumbs in the babies' hair. However, I eat most of my meals and snacks over their heads because they are always nursing, and I am always hungry. Irene doesn't seem to mind the bits of sugar cookie raining down, so long as the milk keeps flowing.

My sister sent me a novelty cookie card. One sugar cookie looks like a chick, the other like an egg. The card is welcome right now. My sugar cravings amp up in the afternoon.

Coming from her, the card is especially poignant. She is in the midst of in vitro fertilization (IVF), and it hasn't been going well. I remember our own experience: the years of low-grade depression—years when time had little meaning for us, each year like the one before except for the increasing aggressiveness of treatment. It seemed like everyone we knew was having children, maturing to the next stage of life, aging naturally. In the mirror, I looked more like a teenager every day. I felt like one. I didn't like it.

When we finally conceived twins via IVF, I was slightly ashamed to fit a stereotype so closely. It felt intemperate to end up with more than one baby. We tried to avoid it, opting for single embryo transfers as long as our contract permitted. To be fair, when we agreed to transfer two embryos, I rooted for both to thrive. My heart quickly wrote new terms of motherhood.

We made it through treatments because I loved my baby for years before she was actually conceived. After a couple years of infertility, I saw an eleven-year-old girl in a play. She had long brown hair like me, was coltish and self-confident. Driving home in the dark, I knew I would have a daughter like her. I loved her already, enough for all the medications to be injected, the miles to be driven, the dollars to be spent. Years later she arrived, one of two embryos.

I did not see a girl with disabilities and intuit that I would some-day be mother to a child like her. Now I must wait to find out who Sallie will be. My heart must revise those terms of motherhood yet again.

THE SUNSET FEED
(tandem)
Irene: Left
Sallie: Right +3 oz
Pump: 4 oz

And now it's getting dark. After this round of pumping, I need to give the pump parts a real washing. Tonight, other people are managing Irene while she screams herself to sleep. Sallie fell asleep at the breast and is peaceful in her bassinet. The pump and I have come to an understanding. I sit and rest while it sings to me. Usually the lyrics are simple:

broccoli, broccoli, broccoli, broccoli.

Or
lollipop, lollipop, lollipop, lollipop, lollipop

Sometimes they are encouraging:

pump lady! pump lady! pump lady! pump lady!

And sometimes the pump philosophizes:

the more you pump, the more you pump, the more you pump, the more you pump

It's almost dark by the time I finish soaking and scrubbing the pump parts. With newborn twins, you develop a new relationship with time. There's the impossible math of breastfeeding one child with a high palate (try to latch thirty minutes, feed at least ten minutes) and another with poor muscle tone (twenty-five minutes), following with a supplemental bottle for both (as long as it takes for each), then pumping milk (ten minutes) and repeating the process again three hours after you started, which is right about when you finish. Day and night cease to have meaning. All times are in this armchair, with this one or that one, napping when possible, in an almost hallucinatory state, opened eyes and closed eyes meaning more than light or dark outside the window.

I used to sleep through every night. I could barely make it through the day on less than eight hours.

THE GLOW WORM FEED
Irene: Right → +1 oz
Sallie: Left +2 oz
Pump: 4 oz

When I'm most fatigued, there is only room in my mind for the most immediate tasks: where is the nipple shield? I found it on the ground earlier and did something with it. I'm so tired. Maybe Sallie will take the nipple bare this time. If I can make it through this feeding, maybe I can skip the start of the next one and leave a bottle for my mother to feed the next baby to wake. I'm covered with milk from a spill during the last pumping. I need to change my shirt. The sash from my sweater coat is missing somewhere. I try to get into the bathroom, but it's locked. I pound on the door. No one is in there. They are all in bed until the next feed. My hands are clutching, shaking. My mom does this all the time, locks the door on one side and exits through the other one. Irene is getting too dependent on the bottle. I don't think she needs it at all anymore. I ought to give her the breast at the next feeding. I tear every cushion off the couch. No nipple shield.

Finally, it turns up on a tray of pump parts. Who put it there? I get the baby latched on, feed her. Swaddle her. Hand her off. The other one. Stumble to the old recliner to sleep.

The house is too full. Jason, the girls. The breast pump. Rotating relatives.

There were eight people in our little room at the hospital, watching while I tried and tried to get Irene to latch, while she screamed, while the lactation consultant soothed. Nurses, relatives, all standing up and craning to get a better look. Get out. Everybody, get out!

What on earth will I do when they go?

THE NIGHT OWL FEED
Irene: Some nursing on Right
Sallie: +3 oz
Pump: 4.5

Even when I fall into deep sleep, I'm aware of the babies, alert to their first cry. Or rather Irene's. She's the one I see and hear in my dreams. She's the one I look for when I wake. Sallie needed bottle feeding more, so others tended her while I held Irene. Sallie is everyone's baby, but I don't really feel that she's mine, not yet. I love Irene passionately and—when she screams for colicky hours—desperately. I love Sallie dutifully.

When she grows up and asks about her babyhood, will I confess?

> *I heard you stirring many nights, but I didn't pick you up or feed you because I knew you wouldn't cry. I fed you last, always, because I knew you would wait until Irene finished. I said to others that this was the gift that you gave us, the way we were able to manage infant twins, but my heart said I was taking advantage of your more passive nature. It wasn't a "gift"; you were the limb I was gnawing off in order to survive.*

But tonight, Sallie wakes and calls out, a crabbed little shout. My still-shrinking uterus cramps with the rush of hormones. I do recognize her, after all. She's learning to fuss, and I will learn to be her mother.

The Feed of Wee Terrors
Irene: Right side-lying giant spit up!
Sallie: +2.5 oz
Pump: 4.5

Sometimes when I'm pumping alone in the dark, the pump's songs take a sinister turn:

> *you pump blood, you pump blood, you pump blood, you pump blood*

Or the paranoid:

> *they are coming, they are coming, they are coming, they are coming.*

I wonder what will happen when I am alone with the girls at last, when our helpers leave. So far, there's no time or solitude for postpartum depression to take root. I've read with interested horror about postpartum psychosis, the rare cases where women go truly mad—some enough to harm their children, to drive them off bridges and drown them in bathtubs.

I read about the attorney who strapped her infant son into a baby carrier and jumped with him off a building. She was morbidly convinced he had suffered brain damage from bumping his head on the carpet and decided to commit double suicide rather than live with a child suffering from a defect. The baby survived the seven-story fall, cushioned by her broken body, although she did not.

I know what form my madness will take, if I ever snap. It will be in the kitchen, the most dangerous room of the house. The new microwave is big enough for a baby. I hide from myself the knowledge of where I keep the hunting knife we use for butchering Muscovy ducks. It horrifies me, but recipes do float into my mind: a simple roast with carrots and potatoes, rosemary and thyme. Irene is fat and tender like a little rabbit, just the right size for the small roaster.

Of course I wouldn't do such a thing, although I do nibble on her darling toes every day in play. I have heard that of the few women who do develop serious postpartum psychoses, only a minute percentage ever hurt their children. But we all have our ideations. Even my grandmother admitted to having the impulse to chuck her crying baby out the open window.

I never imagine eating Sallie.

SUNRISE
Tandem, sequential
Irene: short & sweet, passed out
Sallie: Right ☺
Pump: 4-5 @ 11ish

I dream that we decide to give Irene away to a friend who is infertile. Jason and I walk through the Rockingham County fairgrounds on our way to award her to Becky, but I begin to feel concerned. How could I give up Irene after all? I tell Jason we shouldn't do it. "You should have thought of that earlier," he says. He isn't swayed. It's a relief to wake with the sun in my eyes, knowing that we can keep her. But two still feels like an embarrassing wealth of babies.

The March morning Irene and Sallie were born, I caught a glimpse of each one during the Caesarean, but then went under general anesthesia for the rest of the operation. I truly awoke to the girls a half hour later that morning, my vision doubled as I tried to reconcile what appeared to be two clocks on the wall enough to see whether I had missed a crucial window for establishing nursing. There were two babies, but when my doulas turned back into one doula and the clock resolved into one clock, two distinctly different babies remained.

And then night and day blurred together into the babies' hunger, time floating on an endless stream of milk.

But someday soon, about the three-month mark, time will hook me like a fish, drag me forward, accelerating beyond anything I've experienced. I will find it difficult to snap Irene's yellow romper, the one with the red flowers and the gather in the back that makes her look like a wizened little woman when I sit her up on my lap for a burp. I will realize that it is time to put the romper away, that before a few more moments pass, she'll grow right through the six-month clothes and the 2T's and be in women's eights, towering over me, pitying me for my old-fashioned values, packing her suitcase, out the door, globe-trotting, leaving a great silence in the house.

For a mother coming off three months of evening colic, the prospect of silence should be a considerable relief. But I will panic. The house of my heart has grown new rooms. The twins belong here with us.

I will panic, and then I will be comforted. We have Sallie, too. Sallie, who is just learning to smile, who shouts for joy to see us in the mornings, whose disability or loyalty may keep her at home with us, or at least nearby. With this child, I must let go of my generic aspirations for her, let her define contentment her own way. Nobody knows who she will be or how her potential will change as the world changes. But if she ends up staying close to home, that will be fine with me. And I owe it to Irene to hold her future as lightly as I am learning to hold Sallie's.

I hold them both. I let them go.

Visual Interlude II

6.
Art-i-facts

A Work in Progress

KATHY MANTAS

ARTIST'S STATEMENT

I am a mother of a twin daughter (a twin-less twin or lone twin) and a mother of a twin son who passed away in 2008. In this in-progress art project, I re-explore, re-present, and make meaning of my experience of becoming a mother of multiples through assisted reproductive technologies (ART). In essence, I investigate and share fragments of my story through the use of various personal *ART-i-facts*—created from discards and various items collected from ART procedures.

The broad purpose of this project is to learn more about the fullness of the experience of becoming a mother of multiples through ART. My intent is that *ART-i-facts* will stimulate dialogue about some of the complexities inherent in becoming a mother of multiples through ART (e.g., high-risk multiples pregnancy; surviving traumatic pregnancy and birth experiences; outcomes associated with technological-scientific intervention; mothering multiples; and loss). Additionally, my hope is that *ART-i-facts* will create a safe space for these often silenced stories to emerge as well as to raise questions about the process—both complex and ongoing—of becoming a mother through ART. Moreover, I would like to contribute to ongoing discussions on the value of engaging in more artful approaches to foster more caring medicine.

Finally, this art project also attempts to address the limits of language and text-based discourses and to look more closely at what creative processes and artful approaches have to offer when it comes to making meaning through creative processes and aesthetic approaches; to deepening our understanding of such complex, multilayered, and often (dis)empowering and (dis)mbodied experiences; extending notions of in-fertility and to diversifying maternal representations.

Images are the midwives between experience and language. The miracle of image making … is that it helps birth a story that holds countless memories and emotions. (Malchiodi 24)

INVITATION

I/-*i*- invite you to enter this gathering space and engage directly with the *ART-i-facts*. I bid you to explore and open and close the *ART-i-facts*.

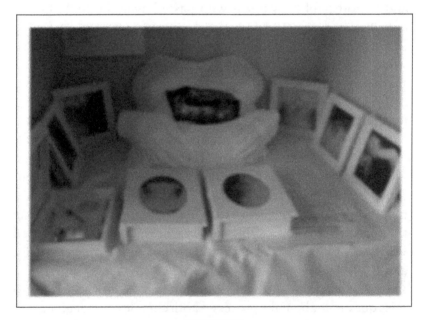

OPENING

There are many ways of telling—"[t]hus, from one telling to the next, our story is not the same, and neither are we" (Lowell Randall 224). For this telling, I choose to begin with the title. In *ART-i-facts*, the "ART" addresses the nature of my artful process—it includes both mixed-media and text-based forms. The "ART" in the title, however, also refers to assisted reproductive technologies.

ART-*i-fact* I

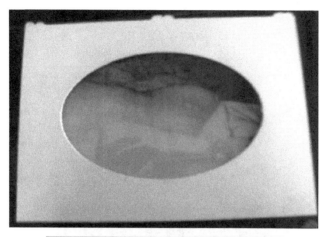

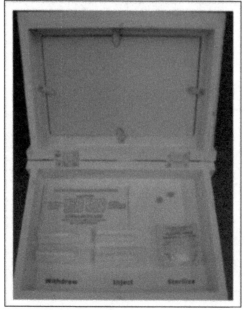

Although there are several others, in-vitro fertilization (IVF) is the most common ART procedure. There are more than a few stages in one IVF cycle: ovarian stimulation, monitoring, and ovulation triggering; egg retrieval; fertilization; and embryo transfer.

ART-i-facts also plays with notions of fact (i.e., scientific facts) and fiction (i.e., artfully crafted forms), especially as they relate to telling and retelling, remembering, and memory. "[M]emory, we are seeing, is really a peculiar brand of fiction, what one psychologist calls 'faction'" (qtd. in Lowell Randall 223).

ART-*i*-fact III

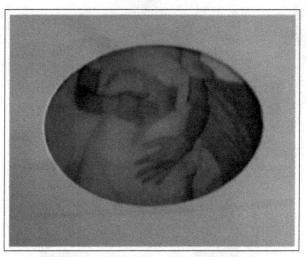

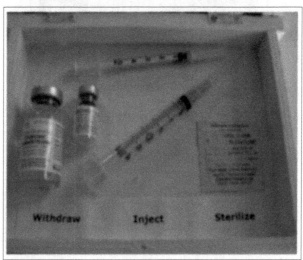

Today, the wide use of fertility drugs and ART procedures such as IVF as well as increased maternal age are considered to be one

of the major contributing factors to the increase in multiple births (Public Health Agency of Canada 31).

I am especially enchanted by the porous quality of memory, and the "eruptions of the past into the present; the way what is gone shapes and shadows what is with us. (Griffin 9)

ART-i-fact III

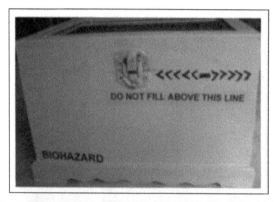

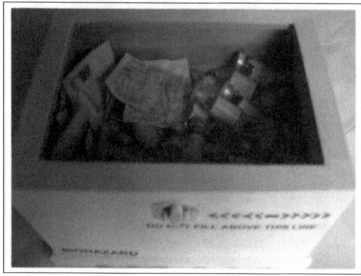

One child in thirteen is a multiple. Over eleven thousand multiple birth babies are born every year in Canada (about 40 percent in Ontario). Between 1997 and 2006, the rate of multiples (per 100

births) increased about 35 percent. Approximately sixty thou-sand multiple birth children of age six and under live in Canada (Launslager).

OPENING FURTHER

In *ART-i-facts*, the *-i-* examines the relationship between my vari-ous subjectivities, which sometimes are in flow, other times are in tension, yet in other occasions are in collision.

ART-*i*-fact IV

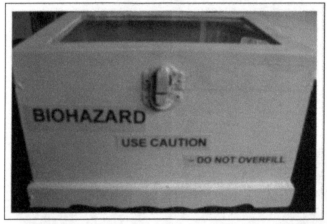

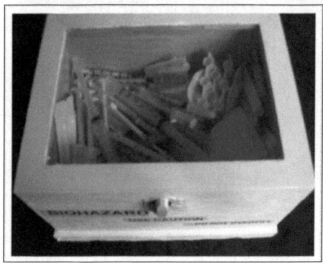

Multiple pregnancies can present significant complications for pregnant women and babies and for mothers, parents, and babies post-birth.

I/-i- am an artist, arts-informed researcher, teacher, daughter, sister, and partner. I/-i- am also an ethnic woman of working-class background and as such, I have always been concerned with issues of knowledge and power. An educated woman of "working class background is among those most likely to be troubled by ... questions [of knowledge and power]. [She] know[s] how radically one can be changed by one's education" (Pagano 44).

ART-i-fact V

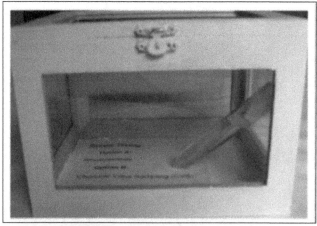

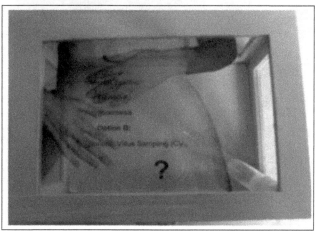

"Multiple births are the fastest growing segment of the preterm birth infant population, representing 20 percent of all preterm births" (Best Start "Low Birth Weight" 4).

I/-*i*- am also an older mother who came to be a mother by way of ART. In *ART-i-facts*, the two dashes around the -*i*- represent being and living in a state of in-betweenness and liminality.

ART-*i*-fact VI

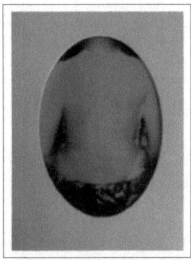

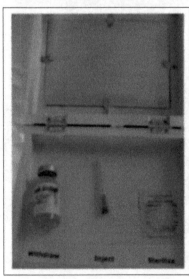

"Infant death is four to five times more likely to occur among multiple births than among singleton births" (Best Start "Low Birth Weight" 4).

This liminal space is "where … women … as creators of literature [and other art forms], … write… [their] own lines, and eventually,…[their] own plays [and stories]" (Heilbrun 102). Although it is a space that is filled with tensions, for me, it is also a creative catalytic opening.

ART-*i*-fact VII

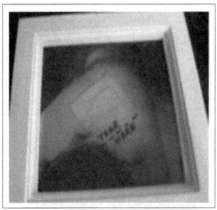

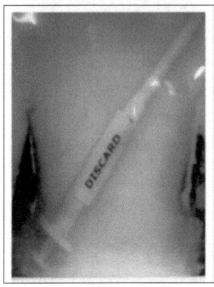

Since death is much higher among multiple births than singletons, parents who lose one, more, or all of their babies face extremely difficult situations (Best Start "Low Birth Weight" 5).

How does one begin to tell of such complex, multilayered and potentially (dis)empowering and (dis)embodied experiences? I choose to tell by creating a multilayered and "multi-voiced" (Lather 9) text, for example, through the use of quotes, repetition of words and *ART-i-facts*.

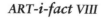

ART-*i-fact* VIII

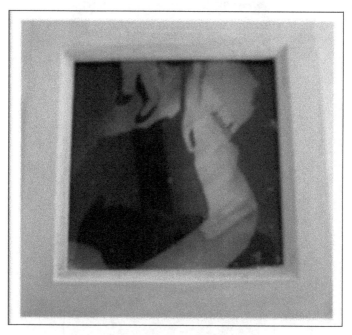

"Medical influence and jurisdiction are most intrusive in the process of childbirth. Here, women must work doubly hard to keep their autonomy and not submit to medicalized rhetoric and opinions (which fails to perceive 'the woman in the body')" (Reis 27).

And I/-i- choose to tell artfully and through paradox. As Palmer states, "Using *and* rather than *but* … expresses a true paradox [italics in original}" (72).

ART-*i*-fact IX

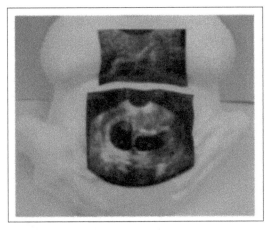

Radical change began with the development of techniques for fetal monitoring (Katz Rothman 157).

I/-*i*- embody paradox, birth *and* death, fact *and* fiction, opening *and* closing, forgetfulness *and* memory.

CLOSING, FOR NOW

And I close, for now, with another story. This story is simply "the story on top at present" (Lowell Randall 338). I/-*i*-am also the daughter of a mother who is a twin. My maternal grandmother, who has passed, gave birth to twins in 1938. My mother has a twin brother.

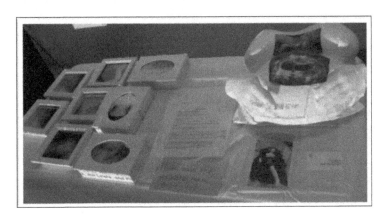

"Yet, it is this second process, composing a life through memory as well as through day-to-day choices, that seems to me most essential to creative living. The past empowers the present, and the groping footsteps leading to this present mark the pathways to the future" (Bateson 34).

I/-*i*- invite you to enter this gathering space and engage directly with the ART-*i-facts*. I bid you to explore and open and close the ART-*i-facts*. And I welcome your comments, suggestions, and questions. Thank you for viewing and participating.

WORKS CITED

Bateson, M. C. *Composing a Life: Life as a Work in Progress—The Improvisations of Five Extraordinary Women*. New York: Penguin Group, 1990. Print.

Griffin, Gail B. *Season of the Witch: Border Lines, Marginal Notes*. Pasadena: Trilogy Books, 1995. Print.

Heilbrun, C. G. *Women's Lives: The View from the Threshold*. Toronto: University of Toronto Press, 1999. Print.

Katz Rothman, B. *Recreating Motherhood: Ideology and Technology in a Patriarchal Society*. New York: W. W. Norton & Company, Inc., 1989. Print.

Lather, Patti. *Getting Smart: Feminist Research and Pedagogy With/In the Postmodern*. New York: Routledge, 1991. Print.

Launslager, Donna. "Helping Families Prepare for Multiple-Birth Children." *Best Start*. Government of Ontario, 2009. Web. 11 Jan. 2015.

Best Start. "Low Birth Weight & Preterm Multiple Births: A Canadian Profile." Toronto: Ontario's Maternal, Newborn, and Early Child Development Resource Centre, 2005. Print.

Lowell Randall, W. *The Stories We Are: An Essay on Self-Creation*. Toronto: University of Toronto Press, 1995. Print.

Malchiodi, C. A. *The Soul's Palette: Drawing on Art's Transformative Powers for Health and Well-Being*. Boston: Shambhala, 2002. Print.

Pagano, J. A. *Exiles and Communities: Teaching in the Patriarchal Wilderness*. Albany: SUNY Press, 1990. Print.

Palmer, P. J. *The Courage to Teach: Exploring the Inner Land-scape of a Teacher's Life*. San Francisco: Jossey-Bass Publishers, 1998. Print.

Public Health Agency of Canada (PHAC). "Canadian Perinatal Health Report," 2008 Edition.

Ottawa: Government of Canada Publications, 2008. Print.

Reis, P. *Through the Goddess: A Woman's Way of Healing*. New York: The Continuum Publishing Company, 1995. Print.

7.
Congratulations and Condolences

Incorporating Burden, Love, and Community in Identifying as a MoM (Or, How I Learned to Stop Worrying and Love the Twins)

ERICA LUCAST STONESTREET

IT IS SURPRISINGLY difficult to explain what defines being a mother of multiples (MoM), other than that it's *more* of everything involved in mothering—work, joy … equipment. Mothering is a challenge, period. Yet given how it feels from the inside, it would be strange to conclude that mothering multiples is not somehow a distinct experience from mothering singletons, even more than one singleton. I started thinking about this as a mother of a singleton and then twins: someone with experience of both should be able to say what the difference is. After much thought and some conversation, I suspect that "more" *is* the defining characteristic of multiple motherhood, but putting it flatly like that doesn't go very far to illuminate the specialness of *MoMhood*.

Unpacking this "more," based primarily on my own experience, I find that three things stand out. Initially salient is the utter burden of infant twins. MoMs often say that "it never ends": somebody always needs you, and somebody's needs are almost always not being met (babies', singleton siblings', partner's, mommy's). For me, burden was the primary experience of mothering multiples for close to eight months. Simultaneously, however, two developments help MoMs cope with the burden and develop themselves *as* MoMs. First, there is the love. Loving multiples requires tremendous work to know and develop several selves at once, including one's own. MoMs commonly say that their capacity to love increases as a result of their multiples. Second, the community of MoMs is a source of comfort and understanding. For example, (in my experience) MoMs are less judgmental of one another and more supportive than other communities of mothers, largely because their views about "correct" methods of mothering are less rigid. They taught me to resist cultural norms of intensive mothering, and that we are "rock stars" just for being MoMs.

Aside from physical exhaustion, perhaps one of the hardest things about expecting and then mothering multiples is being receptive to all three of these elements—burden, love, and community—and using them to grow. Personally, incorporating them into my identity—really *becoming* a MoM—was what got me through those early months, but it was something I had to work at. Nevertheless, the experience provides many opportunities for meaning and, for this reason, can be very rewarding. In the rest of this essay, then, I will argue that multiple motherhood is defined in large part by extra burden, love, and community, that none of these things would be what it is without the others, and that embracing these elements by identifying *as* a MoM is an important step in coping with the challenges. Is this different in kind from the experience of mothering singletons? I'm not certain. But I think the elements interact and intertwine in characteristic and systematic ways that make mothering multiples a distinctive experience.

Let's begin with the burden, but first a confession: I come at this subject from a place of relative privilege. Being a member of the middle class, I don't face the difficulties that less economically privileged mothers inevitably face. Already having a singleton, I was not new to pregnancy or breastfeeding when the twins came along. My twins were spontaneous, my pregnancy had no glitches, not even any hiccups (other than the habitual ones of Baby B), and my girls were born healthy at thirty-eight weeks, four days—full term for twins and well beyond average. Sure, I had a "medicalized" but vaginal birth in the OR (standard procedure for twins), which was not my ideal, but in the end, I was grateful I'd agreed to an epidural. Baby B flipped after her sister made her debut, and she was delivered breech by a funny and competent doctor who was able to reach in and grab her ankle, thus sparing me a C-section. Despite the breech delivery, my experience is nothing compared to the harrowing experiences some mothers of multiples go through, requiring bed rest, the Neonatal Intensive Care Unit (NICU), or both.

I had it easy (on the scale of multiples) after the twins' arrival, too. My husband was unemployed for the last six weeks of my pregnancy and the first six weeks of the girls' lives, and he was an angel through everything. My parents live near enough that they were able to help out almost every day for two months, and for the rest of my leave I had plenty of other help—I never spent a whole day alone with all three of my children until the babies were six months old. I didn't have to learn to feed them without someone there to help me after two weeks, the way many MoMs do; I didn't have to figure out how to entertain my son while I nursed because someone else was almost always there to do it; I didn't have to figure out how to take infant twins and a two-year-old grocery shopping by myself because my own mother was always able to come along. I didn't struggle with postpartum depression. I didn't go back to work until the girls were six months old because they were born in July and, as a professor at a school with relatively decent leave policies, I was able to take a semester off (at reduced pay) to care for them. I didn't even have the minor difficulty of having to learn to tell my daughters apart—they are fraternal, one blond and one brunette.

And yet.

The difficulty of motherhood in general is a kind of open secret that somehow doesn't reach non-parents until it's too late. In mainstream culture, children are portrayed as a joy and a blessing, and even if parents-to-be are told how hard it is to be a parent, they don't truly understand until they're actually parents. In commercials, the difficult things about kids are passed off as minor troubles with simple solutions, fixable with products: diapers, laundry detergent, processed foods, a better refrigerator, or good car insurance. Books like the *What to Expect* series, which contain information on all the things parents might worry about (and some that might not have occurred to them), have an upbeat tone—a willful tenacity with respect to the idea that children are wonderful. This tenacity masks what it really feels like to be exhausted and also the person with ultimate responsibility for this helpless and sometimes unfathomable life. The contrast between the ideal and the reality is present even for mothers of singletons, but it smacks you in the face with multiples. It's not that motherhood is awful.

It's just that its rewards are long term and often subtle—not all joy and giggles and perfect housekeeping—and nothing prepares you for that. Perhaps nothing can. Still, it was not until my twins came along that I used the word "burden" in connection with motherhood.

On the day I learned that our second child was twins, I cried. Not right there in the ultrasound room—I was still shocked—but a little later, in the store where I stopped on my way home to buy a journal for this pregnancy because that was a thing I could do. I cried after dinner that night, before we called all of our family to tell them the news. I recall one relative getting it right when he said, only half-jokingly, "And what's the good news?" I felt this way constantly, almost right up until the girls were eight months old. People would see us in the grocery store and say things like, "Oh, a double blessing! Aren't you lucky!" and many MoMs will tell you that that is not a great thing to say to a mother who is feeling exhausted, frumpy, and burdened. I would paste a grin on my face and say something like, "Not at 2:00 a.m.!" Now my standard response to learning that someone is expecting twins is a heartfelt, "Congratulations!—and condolences." That's all I wanted to hear at that stage, and I was so grateful whenever I encountered someone who understood. Congratulations, you are in an exclusive club with many perks. Condolences, it's a club with steep and ongoing membership dues.

Unlike some mothers, I don't think I felt guilty for not feeling unmixed joy at the news of twins; I knew on some level that it was a perfectly natural reaction. Twins were not in the plan. They meant a lot of extra expense, a zillion comments (sometimes insensitive ones) from strangers, and challenges everywhere you turn. Multiple pregnancy itself is more uncomfortable, exhausting, even disabling. And once they arrive, it is much harder to breastfeed, even if they're good latchers from the start and you learn tandem nursing right away. It is much harder to sleep when "the baby" sleeps, and thus to get enough rest. It is much harder to maintain the household, since every free moment—never mind, there are no free moments for the first few weeks. It is much harder to take twins anywhere because you can only comfort one screaming baby at a time; tandem nursing or bottle feeding is difficult in public;

and getting two babies to sleep in unfamiliar circumstances is near impossible without help. Mothering multiples is much harder emotionally: the moments when you cannot meet every child's needs (let alone yours or your partner's) are far more frequent than they are with singletons, and there is no sense of control and no break. It is hard even with help, because help comes with its own layers of stress: first, feeling dependent on someone for things you used to be able to do yourself; second, even a no-maintenance guest is still someone in your space, doing things not quite the way you'd do them; and third, it's hard not to feel bad handing someone a crying baby, even when that's what she's there to do. The list surely goes on.

Of course, even as I felt this tremendous burden, I knew that at least some of it was the result of my own choices. I didn't *have* to breastfeed the girls; I didn't *have* to be the one to get out of bed every time someone needed feeding or cuddling in the middle of the night and so on. While I was on leave, this was the arrangement that made the most sense; but more than that, oddly, it was what I wanted.

This is what love does for you. One of the hallmarks of love is that it remakes your identity, centring it on the things you love.[1] And it is possible to love a burden. Some burdens are forced on us relational beings arbitrarily, and we must bring ourselves to accept them or be doomed to unhappiness; some are taken up intentionally but may be no less burdensome for that; multiples can be either or both. Love makes it possible to shoulder the burden, to transform an arbitrary situation into an intentional one.[2]

Just as the reality of motherhood is harder and richer than non-parents understand, so too is the reality of love harder and richer than it is often portrayed as being. As I have come to think of it, love is an attitude that picks out a specific person[3] from among the many we encounter and endows him or her with a personal importance beyond the basic, inherent moral importance that all people have. It is *valuative* rather than *evaluative*, we might say. We often say that we love people for their qualities or interests— their sense of humour, their patience, their love of music—and if this is true, then there are many people we *could* love. But there are few we actually do. Because loving is an investment of time

132

and energy that simply cannot be extended to just anyone, it may be somewhat surprising that love is not primarily an evaluative attitude. Something this important might seem like just the sort of thing we would want to screen carefully for. Nevertheless, whom we actually end up loving is partly dependent on external circumstances that have nothing to do with personal compatibility. For instance, the odds of my having the three children I do are staggeringly low. Had things happened just slightly differently, I might have three (or two) very different children from the ones I have. Yet I would love those children just as much as I love the ones I actually have. And although I can compare them to one another and evaluate their different strengths and weaknesses, in *loving* them I simply value them, not evaluate them.

Although love is primarily valuative and not evaluative, it's worth acknowledging the challenges of loving and responding to children as individuals and of aspiring to love them equally (though differently).[4] This is not always easy, given how different children can be from one another and from their parents; multiples bring this lesson home constantly. Loving someone requires seeing her as the person she is and taking an active interest in her interests for her sake. We may love people for their qualities and interests, but we also love their qualities and interests for them.[5] In my son's case, although I do not share his fascination, I have come to a much deeper appreciation of trucks and their great variety than I ever realized was possible. I care about many things because people I love care about them, although some interests are harder to take an interest in than others. Still, as we come to know and to love others, incorporating their interests into our own, they transform from "anyone" to "someone" in our eyes. They become irreplaceable figures in our lives, and we begin to shape our lives in ways that take them into account. Mothering is often cited as a paradigmatic example of love for reasons along these lines: few people will ever know a child as well as his or her mother does, and mothers' lives are shaped to a large extent around their children.

One facet of love that is not often recognized in the context of mothering, or is at least rarely emphasized, is that it is slow to develop. This aspect is easier to recognize in relationships like friendship or romantic love. But although we talk of loving a baby from the start, even before it is born, it has been my experience that love isn't complete until the baby is a few months old. Like most mothers, I was shaping my life around my babies, dedicated to protecting, preserving and caring for them long before they were born. (Eating real ice cream every night in the name of bearing healthy, full-term twins was just one of many sacrifices I made for them.) But love involves seeing another person for who she is, and I couldn't come to truly know—and hence fully love—any of my babies until there was really someone there to know and love; in my experience that takes a few months. Every baby has a unique temperament from the start, of course, and nothing makes this clear like having multiples. (I have one volatile and one mellow twin, which was recognizable right from the first day.) But with all three of my children, although I changed diapers and nursed and rocked and played with them, I didn't feel as if I was interacting with *someone* until a few months had gone by. Perhaps this is part of the burden.

Another facet of love, one that *is* often recognized in the context of mothering, is the way our emotional and volitional investments in those we love make us vulnerable to loss and pain (and joy and pride, let's not forget) that we might not otherwise have been susceptible to. This vulnerability ties our welfare to the welfare of those we love, giving love a somewhat surprising reflexive quality—surprising, given that love is an intrinsically selfless attitude. Here is where the identity element begins to emerge. As my love for my twins deepened and crystallized, I became more and more invested in them as the little people they were, and more and more invested in *being their mother*. I hated all of those 3:00 a.m. wakings, resented being the one to have to get out of bed, and I often felt bored during the day, which meant that the prohibitive difficulty of going anywhere made me feel trapped. Yet at the same time I *wanted* to do the night waking, the daytime playing, and all the rest because I was their mother. Over time, loving them made me receptive to everything mothering them meant (and this is ongoing). Despite all of the struggle, I was (am!) proud of being a good mother to them—one who is attentive and dedicated and does all of these difficult things for her children because she loves them. I was doing the work of caring for them first of all for their sake, of course, but also increasingly for my own sake, because over time, a MoM came to be who I was—even more prominently and deeply than my identity as a mother had been when I had only my singleton. I don't think this would have been the case if it hadn't been for the twins. For me, taking on the extra challenges of twins required letting go of my resentment at the burdens and the lack of control, being receptive to new ways of experiencing and coping with my world, and taking on the identity of a MoM more intentionally than I took on the identity of a mother the first time around. I became a mother when my son was born; I actively embraced and thought critically about the place of mothering in my life when my daughters were born.

I know of MoMs who say that mothering their multiples expanded their capacity to love. The phrase struck me as odd at first, because love is supposed to be something we never run out of[6]—an infinite capacity—and why wouldn't having several singletons do this as well? But if we go beyond a superficial notion of love and focus on what loving a person requires of us, the phrase is not so odd. Love involves attention to another's needs and interests; it involves caring about those needs and interests and working to meet them for that other's sake. And it is not odd to think that we can expand our capacities for attentiveness and work or our capacities for managing the vulnerability that love brings with it. This expansion takes time and is exhausting, particularly with multiples. It can be complicated by things like postpartum depression. And the work of love requires a reshaping of a mother's own identity as someone who does this work and cares this much, at the same time as she works to know and develop the identities of her children. All children have their specific needs, of course. The challenge with multiples is that there are two or more at the same stage of neediness, which is extreme in the first months. You don't have the small advantages of self-sufficiency that even toddlers have by the time a second sibling comes along. And trying to maintain and adjust the partnership with a spouse on top of it all is not an insignificant piece of the challenge.

So far, what I have said sketches a mutual interdependence and reinforcement among the concepts—and experiences—of love, receptivity, intentionality, and identity. It's difficult to say which comes first because they all develop together. I suspect that we sometimes underestimate the magnitude of the adjustment to a new identity that being a mother, and particularly a mother of multiples, involves. Perhaps no one is ever fully prepared for parenthood, but at least with a singleton there are routines and gadgets and plenty of advice. Multiples require a whole new adjustment, and in some small respect, it may be harder for second-time parents because you thought you had it down, and that "bonus baby" pulls the rug out from under you. Routines are much harder to achieve. There is a whole extra set of baby apparatus, a whole extra mouth to feed, another college education to fund, another person to know intimately. A whole new person to *be*—suddenly you have to be the mother of twins or more, someone with twice the infinite patience, twice the tolerance for screaming, and a doubled efficiency quotient. Someone who can manoeuvre a double stroller and a shopping cart while keeping an eye on the walking preschooler. Someone with eyes in the back of her head. Someone with a minivan.

This new identity began to dawn on me well before the girls arrived, of course. (The minivan was one of the first woeful thoughts I had in the ultrasound room.) Even as I struggled with the burdens of bearing and then caring for twins, I simultaneously reveled in the sense of accomplishment and competence, the mommy version of machismo[7] that comes with two infants. While no one understands the burdens like a MoM does, anyone with children knows enough to know that parents of multiples are doing something amazing. Sometime in the first few months, I saw a meme online that said "If God never gives you more than you can handle, God must think I'm a badass." That's how I felt—I was a rock star, because I had to be. (I still tell myself that almost every day.) There were days when all that meant was that everybody was still alive at the end of the day. But hey, I had kept a two-year-old and *twins* alive all day.[8] I was consciously becoming a MoM, and I coped better because of it.

It is difficult and stressful to forge an identity without the support of people in one (or both) of two categories of community: people who share that identity and people who care about you as an individual, thus to some extent sharing your interests. Having both—as I am lucky enough to do—means having understanding from others about the reality that comes with that identity. Understanding breeds support, which makes the identity easier to adopt and live out.[9] In this case, it eases the burden of raising multiples. Community involves sharing, and in particular, I think it involves a shared sense of identity. Shared identity can play out in both types of community.

First, my self-encouragement was helped along when a friend of mine, who became pregnant with twins about six months after I did, added me to a Facebook group for MoMs. This group has been one of the best perks of the whole situation.[10] The MoMs in the group are wise, funny, and supportive. Even though I've never met most of them in person, I'm at home with them in a way that I don't experience with other mothers. There is a solidarity with them that comes from facing a profound challenge and making it through, and it has produced a wonderful sense of community. Contrary to the prominent American cultural myth of the self-sufficient, atomic individual, interaction and interdependence can help people to become and develop who they are.

The women in the MoMs Facebook group share (in the sense of having in common) the direct experience of mothering multiples. With this as a starting point, we come to share (in the sense of give and take) our parenting lessons with one another. This is something I wouldn't have if our second child had been a singleton. Until I had twins, I didn't consciously think of mothering as an activity that needed a support network. Now I realize that this sort of support is what my friends and I had been doing for one another implicitly when our singletons were born. But for me, at least, the support became much more systematic and explicit when I became part of the MoMs group.

The sense of belonging that came with membership in this group helped with the adjustment of my identity. Mothering multiples can be isolating, given the sometimes prohibitive layers of complication it takes to take them anywhere, at least in the early days. The Facebook group connects me with hundreds of other MoMs—enough, in fact, to make it easy to forget that multiples are actually a fairly rare phenomenon. While nursing for forty-five minutes or more at a time, and if I was not reading to my son, I would pull out my phone and check Facebook and would laugh or cry or seek advice or (increasingly, as I became a veteran) contribute my own tips and tricks. Whenever anyone posts a question or just vents about some aspect of mothering multiples, there is an almost immediate chorus of answers and cries of "It gets better, I promise!" Babies' first birthdays are celebrated as an achievement for their mothers. These MoMs sponsor nights out, deliver coffee and meals to the newbies in those first blurry weeks, mourn losses, celebrate births and birthdays, trade clothing and gear, send tips on good or bad activities for kids. These women are great, and I am one of them—someone who is a capable and loving mother, with good days and bad days, just like everyone else. At first, it was simply a tremendous relief to "talk" with other people like me; as time goes on, I find myself identifying more and more with the struggles and joys these other MoMs are experiencing, even though I only know two of them in person.

I'm not the only one who feels this way. A constant refrain in the group is how much people love it. I attribute this to one of the best and also most striking things about this group: the non-judgmental attitude the MoMs take toward parenting decisions. In my experience, MoMs seem to be more tolerant and more united *as* mothers than other groups who bicker about different ways of bringing up children. There is mutual admiration between the stay-at-home MoMs and the MoMs who hold paid jobs; each group recognizes the special challenges the other faces. The paid MoMs honour the stay-at-home MoMs for working just as hard, even though their work is not formally paid or glorified. The stay-at-home MoMs marvel at how the paid MoMs manage a job on top of parenting and a household. It's not this way in the broader culture. There are a number of popular-audience books addressing the rift between the mothers who stay home with their children and those who work outside the home.[11] Each side judges the other for, respectively, not developing their full potential and contributing to the world outside their homes, or not being dedicated enough to their children. The MoMs in my group know that this is nonsense, because different arrangements work for different people and we all develop and fulfill ourselves in different ways. And with multiples, *any* path you choose is hard. Because of this, it is clearer to MoMs that the importance of being united and supported in our common enterprise—raising healthy, happy children—outweighs our interest in evangelizing for (or criticizing for not) doing things according to particular methods or principles.

I am also part of a different parenting group on Facebook, but in contrast to that group, the MoMs understand that when you've got more than one baby or toddler or preschooler, you simply do what you have to do. You've got your parenting principles, but they're flexible with multiples in a way that they don't have to be with singletons. You don't have the luxury of lofty principles when there is more than one running around, chewing on a (hopefully clean) diaper while you're changing the other's. This is not to say that all MoMs agree; we certainly have our differences. But the tone is different. There is less judging and more sharing, more exchange of ideas of what works and what doesn't. We let people do parenting the way that works for them, because that's how it has to be to keep everybody functioning. Sleep in the swing? Absolutely! Kraft macaroni and cheese instead of something organic and/or homemade? Hey, it's quick! "Cry it out" sleep training? A lifesaver. Plunk them in front of the TV now and then? Right on—you have to get a shower. All of these things (and more) would garner at least mild censure in my other mothers' group. The MoMs taught me to lower my expectations of myself (both in parenting and in housecleaning) and to back off from the norms of intensive mothering that it can be easy to get sucked into in middle-class culture. MoMs know that being in control is often out of the question, and they taught me that it's okay.

This was one of the biggest lessons I learned as a MoM. Multiples force parents, early on, to relinquish control in a way they might not otherwise have had to do until the children were much older. One MoM, a friend of mine and mother of two sets of identical twins and a singleton, put it very well:

> [M]ultiples—especially in the early days that stretch parents to their physical limits—stretch the capacity to control, and bring to mind early in parenting the realization that some do not experience until the teen years: "I cannot always

be there. I cannot always fix every problem. I cannot control this process. Should I?"…Certainly people have this realization from other overwhelming life experiences that call for sacrifice for other humans, but with multiples, this experience is almost systematic.[12]

Another MoM in the Facebook group voiced a sentiment echoed by many:

I always tell people that twins make you realize you are not as good of a parent as you think you are. But you also realize you are not as bad of a parent as you think you are! Right off the bat, you see how much genes play a role in temperament and personality, and realize that it's not your job to do something 'the right way' but rather to parent the individuals in the way that best suits them.[13]

Mothers are always nervous about whether we're doing things "right," because we are constantly bombarded by messages glorifying childhood and reinforcing both a maximizing mentality ("Make your child the best!" "Give your child the best!") and an ideal of parenting perfection. But reality is starkly different, and the community that the MoMs in this group experience helps us to resist the pressure to maximize and gives us space to be ourselves.

It's worth clarifying what sort of control is being relinquished here. Parenting a child in the way that best suits her may require control over any number of things[14]—for instance, children with certain kinds of disabilities and sensitivities require special attention to their environment, and even children without disabilities need us to control things like whether dangerous objects are present in their everyday surroundings. Still, the fact that genes do play a significant role in the way children develop should remind us that we must choose what we try to control wisely.[15] "Relinquishing control" in the big picture means relinquishing the maximizing mentality. It calls for worrying less about germs, perhaps, or about what the neighbour's mom is feeding them, or about whether their nap schedules are normal. That is, it calls for less worry about doing things "right."

This suggests a more general point about parenting. Multiples teach those who are immersed in the maximizing mentality that the only way to get through our days is to lower our standards. What this means is not a compromise on what really matters, but *satisficing*—doing well enough—rather than maximizing. And there is research to back up the wisdom of doing so.[16] We should understand that raising multiples doesn't require lowering standards so much as learning to be satisfied with just meeting them and resisting pressure to exceed them. When we examine what truly matters to us—for instance, that the children have enough food, clothing, sleep, and developmental stimulation—we realize that there are many different ways to meet the basic standard, and thus that many different options that might not be acceptable in the maximizing mentality will be acceptable in a satisficing one. So the more general point is that learning to satisfice is important for anyone. Although raising multiples is challenging, period, including for those in a position of privilege, parenting even singletons is difficult. And it is even more difficult for those who lack many of the advantages of middle- and upper-class life. Satisficing can ease some of the stress.

The community of MoMs helped me with big-picture aspects of adjusting to my life as a MoM—and a mom. The second category of community that supports me as a MoM, although I'm well aware that not every MoM has this, is invaluable hands-on local help—in our case, from our family and from our daycare provider. This group has a narrower shared interest: *our* twins. First and foremost, my husband and I became more a team than ever; I am extremely fortunate to have a partner who does his full share of the household and parenting work, and I cannot write an essay about mothering multiples without including him. Similarly, I cannot leave out my own mother. Her involvement in my daughters' care and her interest in my interests (as someone who loves me) have provided support for me *as a MoM* that I am extremely grateful for. I do not do this alone.

In addition to the point I've already made about how sharing interests with others supports identity and thus eases burdens, I can think of two further reasons why identifying myself as a MoM has been key to coping with the difficulty of mothering multiples. These reasons suggest that my experience is not unique. First, embracing the identity of "MoM" helped me to reduce cognitive dissonance. If we find ourselves facing a conflict between our beliefs or attitudes and our actions, we have a tendency to work to reduce that dissonance. In this case, I found myself performing the actions of a MoM, but my attitudes about being a MoM hadn't caught up to these actions. As my love for the girls developed, embracing the identity helped to change the attitudes and reduce the cognitive dissonance. Others who initially greet the news of twins with something less than enthusiasm will probably experience similar cognitive dissonance and will thus likely find identifying as a MoM helpful in reducing it. Second (and relatedly), being *someone who does this* provides a normativity[17] to draw on in difficult moments: since a MoM is who I am, I expect myself to live up to this role, so I hold myself to a standard embodied by it. I thus enable myself to push through without altogether losing patience when we hit the "trifecta" of everyone crying at once. Since we tend to try to live up to the identities we have (or at least those we embrace), again I suspect that I'm not the only one for whom intentionally adopting the identity of MoM will help.

One caveat deserves acknowledgment here.[18] Embracing a "super-MoM" identity without acknowledging the limitations imposed by MoMhood's very real burdens could be devastating rather than empowering. Thinking of MoMs as very capable could have the effect of setting standards much too high and setting ourselves up for failure. Thus, part of my claim in this essay is that the burden is an integral part of the MoM identity, and that part of MoMhood involves recognizing that we are only human; we sometimes fall short because what we're doing is hard.

How different is any of this from what mothers of singletons experience? As I said above, I'm not confident that it's a difference in kind. All mothers can experience burden, love, and community. All mothers can intentionally adopt the identity of mother, and doing so would have the same benefits I've sketched. But I venture to say that the need to do so is more urgent with multiples. The initial heavy burden imposed by multiples, and the way love and community can develop around it—and consequently help to ease it by making the identity of MoM easier to adopt—are more systematic for mothers of multiples than they are for mothers of singletons. Because of the burden, MoMs may have to work harder to be receptive to their roles. Drawing on the resources of love and community can help with this receptivity, creating a virtuous circle that makes success in incorporating their motherhood into their personal identities more likely. The way these three elements intertwine in the "more" of MoMhood gives the experience of mothering multiples the distinct character it has. Identifying as MoMs, in turn, helps to reinforce the circle and ease the burdens, or at least cope with them. This is the main message I would give to any new MoM, along with my congratulations and condolences.

As time goes on, I find myself assimilating the new normal. The sense of the whole thing being so hard is starting to fade. The burden is lessening. Whether this is because it really is getting easier or because I have simply acclimated I can't clearly say—no doubt it's both. The twins have become a real source of joy for me; I no longer see twins as the very mixed blessing that was my primary experience for so many months. That feeling is one I don't want to forget, although I'm glad to be past it. The burden and the struggle are a central part of who I am now, but they are bearable because of love's mitigating force and community's support and reassurance—neither of which would be what they are without the burden. Teaching Camus's "Myth of Sisyphus" this past spring, I realized that I feel very much like Camus's reimagined character: my rock is my thing. In the Greek myth, Sisyphus was condemned by the gods to roll a rock up a mountain every day, only to have it roll back down every night. This is supposed to be a terrible punishment because of the utter futility and meaninglessness of his task. My task is far from futile or meaningless, of course, but on some days, it does feel as though the work is going nowhere. No matter how many diapers you change, the next one will get soiled; no matter how much you clean, messes rematerialize; no matter how often you feed, hunger returns. It is hard work. But on Camus's interpretation, Sisyphus transcends his fate by scorn, making it meaningful by owning it: he becomes (in his own mind, at least) the best damn rock pusher the gods have ever seen. His rock is his thing, as

Camus puts it. Like this reimagined Sisyphus, I embrace my fate by identifying with my mothering work. But there is no scorn here; instead there is love and community. Mothering is what I do now. It's who I am. To paraphrase Camus, one must imagine a MoM happy.

NOTES

[1]For extensive philosophical discussions of this attitude, see Helm, Frankfurt ("Final Ends" and "Reasons"), Jaworska, and Anderson. With the exception of the later Frankfurt, these sources employ the word "care" for what I am calling "love," but I choose the latter term in order to distinguish the attitude from the activity of caring, although, of course, the two are closely intertwined. My philosophical understanding of love is also indebted to Velleman ("Love" and "Beyond Price") and, broadly speaking, the work of Irving Singer.
[2]I thank Dennis Beach for the "arbitrary vs. intentional" language here.
[3]For purposes of this essay, I'll limit my discussion of love to persons. I believe it can also be useful to talk about love of "projects" in a broad sense, such as hobbies or causes that people pour themselves into, but in the current context this merely adds unnecessary layers to the discussion.
[4]Thanks to Donna Engelmann for reminding me of this.
[5]Thanks again to Dennis Beach for this point.
[6]"Supposed to be something we never run out of"—this is a stereotype about love, and like all stereotypes, it has its limitations. It is possible for love to be stretched too far. But this is not the place to pursue this thought.
[7]Although "machismo" has connotations of looking down on and even denigrating women, I've decided it's not too much here. I find myself with, and occasionally detect in other MoMs, a slight attitude of proud (though mostly good-natured) superiority over singleton mothers.
[8]This comment is not intended to hurt or even judge mothers who have suffered the loss of a child. Losing a child does not in the least entail subpar mothering. The comment is the expression—not

unique to me—of how some mothers look for a silver lining at the end of a trying day.

[9]We see this in the push to recruit people from under-represented groups into positions of prominence in government, popular culture, corporate management and entrepreneurship, science and math, and so on. The hope is that once there are well-known role models, it will become easier for others to follow in their footsteps, and eventually make the demographics of all of these areas match those of the wider population.

[10]While the Facebook group is a virtual community, it is no less a community. Its virtuality may be an advantage because it grants access to social connections for many more people than may have had it before the Internet age, and it is available even when you can't get yourself and your children out the door, thus easing the isolation of MoMhood. Still, community is not a universal experience for MoMs, so I can't claim that it is always a defining aspect of MoMhood in the same way that burden and love likely are. Nevertheless, community has been integral to and definitive of mothering multiples for me, and I'm confident that others share this experience—and did so before the advent of the Internet, although it may have been harder then.

[11]See, for instance, Steiner and Peskowitz.

[12]Comment on author's Facebook post in Minneapolis Mamas with Multiples Facebook group. Web. 4 June 2014. Name removed to preserve anonymity.

[13]Comment on author's Facebook post in Minneapolis Mamas with Multiples Facebook group. Web. 4 June 2014. Name removed to preserve anonymity.

[14]I thank Sarah Buss for pointing this out.

[15]Thanks to Sara Protasi for highlighting this.

[16]See Schwartz.

[17]"Normativity" in the philosophical sense: prescriptive rather than descriptive. Identities are normative for us because they set up ideals. This idea can be found in various places: Korsgaard is a prominent example; Velleman ("Ideal"); Appiah (see especially p. 24-6); also Frankfurt, Anderson, and Helm.

[18]I'm grateful to Donna Engelmann for pointing out this cautionary note.

WORKS CITED

Anderson, Elizabeth. *Value in Ethics and Economics*. Cambridge, MA: Harvard University Press, 1993. Print.

Appiah, Kwame Anthony. *The Ethics of Identity*. Princeton: Princeton University Press, 2007. Print.

Frankfurt, Harry. "On the Usefulness of Final Ends." *Necessity, Volition, and Love*. New York: Cambridge University Press, 1999. 82-94. Print.

Frankfurt, Henry. *The Reasons of Love*. Princeton: Princeton University Press, 2004. Print.

Helm, Bennett W. *Love, Friendship, & the Self: Intimacy, Identification, & the Social Nature of Persons*. New York: Oxford University Press, 2010. Print.

Jaworska, Agnieszka. "Caring and Internality." *Philosophy and Phenomenological Research* 74.3 (2007): 529-68. Print.

Korsgaard, Christine. *Sources of Normativity*. New York: Cambridge University Press, 1996. Print.

Peskowitz, Miriam. *The Truth Behind the Mommy Wars: Who Decides What Makes a Good Mother?* Berkeley, CA: Seal, 2005. Print.

Post. *Facebook*. Facebook, 4 June 2014. Web. 4 June 2014.

Schwartz, Barry. *The Paradox of Choice: Why More is Less*. New York: HarperCollins, 2004. Print.

Steiner, Leslie Morgan. *Mommy Wars: Stay-at-Home and Career Moms Face off on Their Choices, Their Lives, Their Families*. New York: Random House, 2007. Print.

Velleman, J. David. "Beyond Price." *Ethics* 118.2 (2008): 191-212. Print.

Velleman J. David. "Motivation by Ideal." *Philosophical Explorations* 5.2 (2002): 90-104. Print.

Velleman J. David. "Love as a Moral Emotion." *Ethics* 109.2 (1999): 338-374. Print.

8.
Surviving the Early Years

Parents of Multiples' Trials and Tribulations of Finding and Accessing Suitable and Affordable Childcare

JENNIFER KELLAND AND ROSE RICCIARDELLI

FINDING ACCESSIBLE, AFFORDABLE, and suitable childcare (e.g., licensed or in-home child minding for infants, toddlers, and children) is challenging in most Canadian provinces. Furthermore, in some regions, childcare costs are more than a third of mothers' salaries (Nguyen), and spaces in licensed childcare programs are limited—even unoffered until a child is eighteen months or older. In 2006, Canadian childcare systems placed last among the Organization for Economic Co-Operation and Development (OECD) countries when ranked on the accessibility of quality early childhood care and education (Amoroso). Perhaps this fact is reflected in Canada's lack of a universal childcare program, despite offering a Universal Child Care Benefit (UCCB) that provides $100 (Canadian currency) per month per child age six or younger for childcare (Holland). Conversely, some argue that this program provides minimal financial support to families *and* fails to recognize the need for universally accessible childcare options (Amoroso).

Regardless of tax credits, childcare costs are central considerations for families when deciding whether both parents will work, given childcare is primarily sought to assist parents in meeting their work demands. A second, closely related, consideration is the cost of childcare versus the income provided by employment. Immervoll and Barber indicate that childcare costs are invaluable in determining the financial benefits of working with young children. In some situations, parents cannot afford to work after having children, since their earnings only, or do not even, cover their childcare costs. Moreover, as McKinley argues, Canadian women may choose childcare providers or services based on its availability and cost rather than childcare desires, which often results in the use of unlicensed day-home or in-home daycare programs that bring instability and unpredictability. This leaves mothers seeking last-minute alternative care options much too often. Prentice ("Childcare, Co-production, and the Third Sector in Canada") argues that the current system of childcare provision results in "parent-controlled" childcare centres that place additional demands on families, particularly mothers. Clearly, childcare decisions are largely based on costs and availability (Davis and Connelly).

USE OF CHILDCARE

Most Canadian families have access to some paid maternity leave and parental leave during their first year postpartum, although parents of multiples have been unable to access dual parental leave (MBC, "Supreme Court of Canada Decision"). Since parents are eligible for 35 weeks of parental leave between them (if their occupation permits the option), they often turn to other family members and friends to provide childcare during this first year. In families with multiples, the need for childcare is fundamental to provide required basic care to infants. For example, caring for six-month-old triplets takes an average of 197.5 hours each week—impossible given there are only 168 hours in a week. Thus, one parent cannot care for these babies alone, let alone take time to care for him or herself as well (Best Start "Low Birth Weight").

With increasing needs for dual-income families, alongside increasing rates of multiple births, the demand for childcare is escalating. A recent Canadian study by Sinha noted that more than 60 percent of families with children between the ages of two and four used childcare, and over 71 percent of households with two working parents and 58 percent of lone-parent families used childcare for preschool-aged children. Demand for childcare, as predicted, was lowest among families in which only one parent worked (42 percent) or for children under 1 year of age because of maternity and parental leave employment benefits—however, this need continues to exist and remains unmet (Sinha).

TYPES OF CHILDCARE

Childcare refers to "non-parental care, that is, the care of children by someone other than a parent or guardian" (Sinha). Childcare then does not necessarily involve payment and can be provided by extended family or siblings who do or do not receive financial contributions. Among preschool childcare options, Sinha has developed three categories of care in Canada: "daycare centres, home daycares and private arrangements, such as grandparents, other relatives or nannies." Once children are in formal elementary schooling, before and after school programs constitute an additional form of childcare.

In Canada, childcare services are regulated by provincial and territorial governments. Each province determines the regulations for identifying registered or regulated childcare services that, typically, can be used to access grants and financial benefits (e.g., funding available to support childcare offered by family members in select provinces). Unregulated services, however, are not recognized and do not qualify for any funding. Prentice ("Less Access, Worse Quality") highlighted that only one in seven children had access to regulated childcare, and it was often families from lower socio-economic groups that found their access to regulated childcare limited—thus starting the processes of stratifying children by socio-economic gradients prior to starting school.

CHILDCARE FOR MULTIPLES

A lacuna exists in the literature on childcare as pertaining to families with multiples. Few researchers—such as Robin, Corroyer, and Casati in France—have highlighted the demands tied to caring for multiple children, with an emphasis on mothers as care providers in the first year. They have found that after the initial stage of infant care parents provide, very limited research exists on how parents arrange childcare.

In the United Kingdom, McKay found that families of multiples were more likely to rely on their partners: 46 percent of families with multiples, in comparison to 30 percent of those with singleton(s), relied on their partners for care and families of multiples were less likely to have access to private childcare centres (11 percent versus 18 percent) or a babysitter (11 percent versus 15 percent). Families with multiples were more likely to hire a nanny or au pair in comparison to families with one or more singleton children (14 percent versus 3 percent). Families of multiples, in McKay's study, relied on an average of 1.6 methods of childcare, confirming that childcare arrangements often involve multiple solutions and, as expected, costs of childcare are higher for families with multiples. Researchers have also found that mothers of multiples to be less likely to return to work nine months after their babies were born (MacKay), and that their level of workforce participation—as found by researchers in Australia (Fisher) and the United Kingdom (Glazebrook et al.)— has remained lower than average, even up to 18 months postpartum. Furthermore, researchers have shown that mothers of multiples are more likely than those of singletons to plan not to return to work until their children are in school fulltime (MacKay).

METHODS

The Twins and Multiple Birth Association (TAMBA) in the United Kingdom, in partnership with Multiple Births Canada (MBC), conducted an online survey of families of multiples. Although the survey was developed by TAMBA, members of MBC's Health and Education Committee and the MBC executive committee reviewed the survey suggesting revisions in wording and content to adapt the survey for Canadian respondents. The survey was available online between December, 2013 and February, 2014. Participants were recruited by MBC and affiliated local organizations that support families of multiples by advertising the study through their organizational newsletters and social media. Approximately 80 percent (*n*=77) of the respondents indicated that they were members of a local multiples organization and/or MBC. Inclusion criteria comprised two factors: participants must have multiples (two or more children born from one pregnancy) and must be the primary caregiver for their multiples.

The survey included 61 questions to garner information on family structure, childcare situations and costs, parents' employment status, and the family's financial situation. Preliminary descriptive data is reported here, largely frequencies.[1] Open-ended data are included to provide context to the quantitative data. Any direct quotes are minimally edited for grammar, flow, and clarity.

PARTICIPANTS

The majority of the respondents are biological mothers of multiples in their 30s (68 percent), with fewer over age 40 (23 percent)—again reflecting the increasing number of multiple births among older women (who are more likely to have multiples than younger women due to biological factors affecting fertility [Hankins and Saade]). Furthermore, the majority of respondents lived in urban centres (84 percent, n=78) with fewer in rural areas (18 percent, n=17).[2] Table 1 provides complete respondent demographic information; missing data are removed.

Participants were mothers of twins (89 percent, n=233), or higher order multiples such as triplets or quadruplets (12 percent, n=31). Beyond their multiples, 35 percent (n=92) also had another single-ton child, and 12 percent (n=32) have two or more non-multiple children. Two respondents had more than one set of multiples, and three respondents were expecting twins. The average number of children per family was 2.8. Children's ages were fairly evenly divided into six categories (see Table 2).

RESULTS

The survey results are presented first by describing how respondents use childcare in their families, followed by how they select a childcare provider, and finally by their reasons for using and not using childcare. Next, three themes in the research are explored: cost, availability, and suitability.

CHILDCARE USE IN FAMILIES WITH MULTIPLES

Biological mothers who are primarily making childcare decisions in families with multiples overwhelmingly report (75 percent, n=199) using childcare. This level of use is higher than the Canadian average,

Table 1

Survey Respondents Demographics for Childcare Survey

	Response Percent	Response Count
Person who completed the survey (n=266)		
Mother	99.9%	264
Partner - Female (not the biological mother)	0.7%	2
Age (n=266)		
20-29	9.1%	24
30-39	68.0%	181
40 or over	22.9%	61
Location (province or territory in Canada) (n=266)		
Alberta	15.4%	41
British Columbia	9.8%	26
Manitoba	1.1%	3
New Brunswick	1.9%	5
Nova Scotia	0.8%	2
Nunavut	0.4%	1
Ontario	62.4%	166
Quebec	0.8%	2
Saskatchewan	7.5%	20
Location (urban/rural) (n=99)		
Urban	83.9%	78
Rural	18.3%	17
Other	2.2%	4

as shown by Sinha to be 60 percent. Furthermore, respondents' open-ended comments reveal that some participants who stated they did not use childcare actually did and should be added to the reported 75 percent, which would suggest that childcare use is higher than reported: "I rely on my sister since childcare is too expensive and I will have to quit my job when she goes back to work from her own maternity leave" (Participant 1).

On average, participants used 2.1 types of childcare. Although consistent with MacKay's findings in Britain that families tend to use more than one type of childcare, our findings suggest that

Table 2
Ages of Children in the Respondent's Family (n=266)

	Response Percent	Response Count
0-12 months	23.3%	62
12-24 months	25.9%	69
2-3 years	24.4%	65
3-4 years	23.6%	63
4-5 years	22.9%	61
6-12 years	25.1%	67
13-18 years	4.5%	12
18+ years	3.0%	8

* Note that some respondents provided more than one response.

Canadian families of multiples use more forms of childcare than families of multiples in the United Kingdom. Thus, families rely on full-time and part-time childcare solutions, including care by family members (grandparents, siblings, other family members), in-home care (nanny, au pair, babysitter), daycares and day homes, educational programs (preschool, nursery school) and before and after school care. They used registered or regulated options, and private childcare solutions to meet their needs (e.g., most care provided by family, nannies, and babysitters would be considered unregulated) (see Table 3).

SELECTING A CHILDCARE PROVIDER

Sinha, in her Canadian study, identified location as the top reason for choosing childcare (33 percent), followed by trusting the childcare provider (18 percent), affordability (11 percent), and, as a participant stated, "feeling that it was the only option available" (11 percent) (7). Among our participants, location was the primary reason for mothers to elect to use a specific childcare provider (84 percent, n=81), closely followed by the provider's qualifications (79 percent, n=77) (see Table 5). However, the overwhelming majority of respondents were concerned about the availability of spaces for multiples and their siblings (70 percent, n=67).

Table 3
Types of childcare Used by Families (n=159)

	Response Percent	Response Count
Daycare Centre	36.3%	57
Grandparent	35.7%	56
In-home Daycare	26.8%	42
Babysitter (paid, after hours)	24.2%	38
Other Family Members	17.8%	28
Nanny (live in or live out), Nurse, Au Pair	15.9%	25
Private Day Home	14.0%	22
Friends	12.7%	20
After School Programs	10.8%	17
Registered Day Home	5.1%	8
Preschool, Montessori School, Nursery School, Camp	4.5%	7
Drop-in Childcare	2.5%	4
Older Siblings	2.5%	4
Mothers' Day Out Programs	1.3%	2
Workplace Daycare	0.6%	1

*Note that some respondents provided more than one response.

REASONS FOR NOT USING CHILDCARE

Mothers who elected not to use childcare cited cost as the main deterrent (68 percent, n=45). Specifically, the cost of childcare for multiples was thought to be higher than their monthly earnings. One participant, for example, said, "I stayed home for eight years, too expensive for two toddlers that were not potty trained, my whole pay—plus $30—was going towards childcare" (Participant 2). Thus, despite mothers reporting that they would have liked to use daycare—"[we] would put the twins in a few days each to learn to socialize and get a break from each other" (Participant

Table 4
Factors that Influence Choice of Childcare (n=97)

	Response Percent	Response Count
Proximity to Home	83.5%	81
Qualifications of Childcare Workers	79.4%	77
Available Places for Multiples and/or Other Siblings	69.1%	67
Philosophy of Childcare	56.7%	55
Lunches and Snacks Provided	54.6%	53
Proximity to Workplace of Either Partner	48.5%	47
Educational Component	48.5%	47
References or Referrals from Friends or Families	47.4%	46
Number of Other Children	46.4%	45
Part-Time or Flexible Scheduling Options	37.1%	36
Extended Hours	37.1%	36
Before and After School Care	30.9%	30
Approved Program for Government Grants	27.8%	27
Size of Program	22.7%	22
Proximity to Children's Schools	21.6%	21
Discounts for Families of Multiples	18.6%	18
Transportation to School Provided	11.3%	11
Accessible by Public Transport	3.1%	3
Religious Affiliation	2.1%	2
Other **	3.1%	3

*Note that some respondents provided more than one response.
**Other responses: 1. Experience with Multiples; 2. Treat My children like Their Own; 3. Any Place with Space, No Matter How Far.

3)—the high cost eliminated the option as well as the lack of available childcare (14 percent, *n*=9). Mothers who reported not needing childcare (38 percent, *n*=25) often chose to stay home: "I'm the mother, I raise my own, not someone else" (Participant 4). These mothers tended to recognize the benefits of their financial position as they had the needed funds to do so: "[I'm] fortunate to be able to live off of one income and enjoy time with them until school begins" (Participant 5). This group included a select few mothers who had the financial flexibility to choose to stay home with their children.

REASONS FOR USING CHILDCARE

Childcare was primarily used to enable mothers to return to work (90 percent, *n*=160), although some reported using care to provide mothers with some free time (33 percent, *n*=58) or to assist with providing immediate care for other children, specifically when they needed to take a child to a medical appointment (15 percent, *n*=27). Indeed, mothers of multiples required additional childcare simply to meet the care needs of their other children. Multiples are more likely than singleton children to have medical needs (MBC, "Multiple Births Facts and Figures"), which presents additional significant childcare challenges for mothers of multiples (see Table 6).

On average, respondents used 59 hours of childcare per week during the school year, with a median of 40 to 49 hours per week (21 percent, *n*=36). Since these families have an average of 2.8 children, these numbers suggest that most children were receiving part-time care, which could include a number of different childcare arrangements. For example, preschool twins in part-time care plus an older sibling in afterschool care, or three children in before and after school care, or a singleton infant in childcare and school-age twins not in childcare could be potential childcare arrangements. Another 28 percent of families (*n*=50) used between 10 and 39 hours per week, and 28 percent (*n*=48) used between 70 and 109 hours per week, with 109 hours per week equating to nearly full-time (38.9 hours) care for an average of 2.8 children.

Table 5
Reasons for Using Childcare (n=175)

	Response Percent	Response Count
To Enable Me to Work	90.9%	159
To Enable Me to Have Some "Free" Time	32.6%	57
To Take One or More Children to Medical Appointments	15.4%	27
To Attend School, Study, or Conduct Research	5.7%	10
To Volunteer	5.1%	9
Because It Is Offered Free by the Government/Employer/Other	2.3%	4
To Look for Work	2.3%	4
To Have More Time with Children	2.3%	4
To Care for Family Members Other Than Children	1.7%	3
Socializing, Development, Time with Other Children	1.7%	3
Self-care	1.7%	3
To Do Errands	1.7%	3
Recovering from Injury	0.6%	1
"To Meet Their Needs since Birth"	0.6%	1

*Note that some respondents provided more than one response.

During school holidays, families used slightly fewer hours of childcare per week (52). However, 20 percent (n=34) of families did not use childcare during holidays, which was likely a result of approximately 20 percent (n=34) of wage earners in our sample being employed in the field of K-12 education. Furthermore, during the holidays, a greater number of families used more than 120 hours of childcare (n=18, 10 percent compared to 9 percent, n=15) with families using up to 279 hours of childcare per week, which suggests that school-aged children also require full-time care during the holidays. Thus, although overall childcare needs are reduced during school holidays, they remain prevalent with some families requiring significantly more care. Furthermore, recognizing that some termination of childcare use during holidays is the result of daycare-childcare facilities being closed or on reduced hours, it is impossible to know how much of the reduction in care needs is indicative of reduced needs versus reduced availability.

THEMES

The three predominant themes—affordability, availability, and suitability—prevailed as issues identified by respondents in finding childcare. Affordability includes overall costs as well as how childcare corresponds with work and other related childcare needs. Availability includes the possibility of finding space(s), and how much time is spent on waitlists to access childcare, whereas suitability includes finding childcare that meets the specific needs of families of multiples, including scheduling, the quality of childcare, and any other criteria required of the childcare provider.

AFFORDABILITY

Childcare costs consumed a large portion of a family's income, with 31 percent (n=49) of participants spending up to 10 percent of their household income on childcare; 28 percent (n=44) spending 11 to 20 percent; and 30 percent (n=47) spending between 21 and 40 percent of their annual income on childcare. The average annual childcare cost per family in this study—which may include full or part-time preschool childcare and/or before and after school care of older children—was reported as $17,237, slightly less than the cost of singleton full-time infant care in Toronto, which is just over $20,000 per annum (Noakes). Thus, participants were paying a lot for the provision of minimal childcare. In cases of childcare for multiple infants the costs were considerably higher: "Fulltime childcare for triplets is more than I made" (Participant 6) and "It is expensive. If we were not a two-income family we would never be able to afford it" (Participant 7). Furthermore, the childcare costs affected their overall life choices and quality of life, as some elected not to have additional children in light of the extra child-care costs that they simply would not have been able to afford: "We would like to have more children. But unfortunately with the cost of childcare and because of our salaries we do not qualify for any financial assistance from the government. We are comfortable financially but if we had one more, daycare costs for three fulltime children would outweigh everything else" (Participant 8). Another participant explained that

> We would love to buy a bigger home, however, we haven't been able to save over $175,000. We have to dip into our savings once and a while due to ongoing expenses. My one twin recently was hospitalized and I missed a lot of work.... We go away for one week to a rustic cottage—we can't afford all-inclusive vacations like we once enjoyed before having kids.... Our kids attend two recreational activities a week—I would love for them to take music and swimming too but we can't afford that right now to. (Participant 9)

As evidenced in these excerpts, mothers reported being unable to upgrade or purchase a new home or vehicle or other such luxuries as their money was tied up in childcare needs.

In this study, for families with three or more children requiring childcare, daycare was often expensive and difficult to access. As one mother pointed out, a nanny is a cost-effective alternative, but this solution presents other challenges: "For higher-order-multiple families the most cost-effective childcare is often hiring a nanny to come in to the home or live with the family—but they are difficult to find and hire, and don't always work out well. (I've heard stories from friends with larger families)" (Participant 10). Moreover, the fact that multiples are often "surprises" creates an additional financial challenge for families who have little time to prepare for the costs of multiples, particularly given childcare costs are directly linked to work. Moreover, saving is nearly impossible when on sick, maternity, or parental leave. One participant explained it in the following way:

Many singleton pregnancies are planned for, many multi-ple-foetus pregnancies are not. One cannot plan for double the childcare cost well in advance. You have 18 years to plan for double the cost of university education. Less than 3 years for double the cost of childcare. And which costs more? ... [having twins] certainly continues to present financial difficulties, particularly in the area of childcare. (Participant 11)

Although 35 percent (*n*=52) of respondents received some contri-butions to help with childcare costs, usually in the form of UCCB, such contributions for 48 percent of respondents (*n*=24) covered less than 10 percent of their total childcare costs. Less than a quar-ter of families received a minimal discount for enrolling multiples (and their siblings) in full-time childcare (rarely, if the children were enrolled part time). Such discounts were minimal: "We get a discount of about $50 per month" (Participant 12); "5 percent for the second child" (Participant 13); "We are saving a total of $105 for 3 kids" (Participant 14); or "She just gave me about $10 off the whole bill per week" (Participant 15). As evidenced above, the discounts were rather small.

As previously noted, childcare costs affected whether both parents in a two-parent family work after the birth of multiples. Although only five percent (*n*=9) of respondents indicated the main wage earner stopped working because of childcare costs, 25 percent (*n*=43) reported that the "other" parent—the secondary wage earner—did not return to work. In all but one case, respondents' comments suggest that the mother terminated her employment to care for the children. Yet having only one parent employed often meant that the employed parent worked additional hours to financially support the family: "He works more than 18 hours a day even on weekends to help cover our costs" (Participant 16). In fact, 56 percent of main wage earners (*n*=112) were working more than 41 hours per week. Even with working additional hours, the family tended to experience some financial difficulty. One participant stated, "I stopped working and became a stay at home mom and I struggle each month" (Participant 49). Others found alternative ways to save money while staying home as this participant explained, "for me to stay home, we continue to rent" (Participant 17). Of course, many respondents stopped working completely because of the cost of childcare, although in some cases the mother wanted to stay home and welcomed the justification (e.g., "I wanted to stay home, but the cost of twins in daycare in Toronto is a huge expense, so that helped justify our decision" [Participant 18]). Unsurprisingly, respondents on maternity leave were also considering not returning to work postpartum. One woman said, "I am on maternity leave now and may not be able to go back if I can't find space or affordable daycare for my three girls" (Participant 19), whereas another said, "I'm on maternity leave and had to cancel our daughters' daycare due to costs" (Participant 20). As evidenced here, costs remained a major obstacle for childcare for these mothers. However, despite the costs, some mothers returned to work for the long-term benefits:

> Childcare is expensive, but I also know that I have a pension with the company I work with. The dilemma for us when my maternity leave was up was that my husband is a trade worker. He cannot always find work and that I was not prepared to throw away my pension. I don't want to be a burden on my children when I have to retire. It is a big issue of scrimp now to prepare for later. (Participant 21)

These mothers tended to avoid a challenge that many who stay at home when their children are young eventually face—the inability to find suitable employment after their children are in school full-time. For example, a respondent explained that she stayed home when it was cost effective; however, she found returning to work difficult:

> I recently went back to work, but couldn't find a job in my field—despite previous experience and education—because the experience was not recent. Affordable childcare back then would most likely have kept my skills current. I am starting over, working with college-age students, while my peers are in better positions. Coincidentally, my peers have all had singleton children. (Participant 22)

As her words suggest, her career was negatively impacted by her decision to stay home, which may explain by the secondary wage earner, often the mother, terminated her employment to provide childcare, while the primary wage earner continued working.

AVAILABILITY

Finding childcare spaces for multiple children was a challenge for many participants (63 percent, n=81). Beyond the 14 percent (n=9) of participants who did not use childcare due to its unavailability, nearly half (47 percent, n=101) of the families using childcare had been on waitlists prior to obtaining placements. Respondents reported that this was often a result of provincial regulations restricting the number of childcare spaces allowed for infants in private day homes or in-home daycares to two per location. For a family with twins, in this study, finding a location with two infant openings was very difficult. Participants stated finding spaces for twins was challenging: "regulations only allow 2 kids under 2. This limits spaces, as I won't separate my twins" (Participant 23). Families with triples faced even greater challenges: "it was impossible to find an in-home daycare with room for infant triplets" (Participant 10). This difficulty was compounded by the fact that many families also required care that accommodated the siblings of their multiples (e.g., "[I was] unable to get 1 infant and 2 toddler spots to open up at the same time" [Participant 25]). This situation not only required having more childcare spaces available but also highlighted another challenge: caring for multiples, particularly young multiples with singleton siblings or higher order multiples, can be intimidating for a sole childcare provider.

Indeed, a common concern here was the mother's desire to not "separate" children to acquire care. Thus, to secure placement, many families placed their children on one or more waiting lists— even unborn children: "I was on around 7 wait lists since I was 15 weeks pregnant. My children are currently 13 months old and I have not heard from any daycare yet" (Participant 26). Another participant echoed this strategy: "When I was pregnant I placed my unborn twins on a waitlist for when they would turn 18 months. I was first (and second) on the list. It turns out that I will not enroll them until they are 26 months" (Participants 27). These excerpts display the realities of waiting for childcare and that even signing up for care when pregnant does not ensure future placement. This was clearly a genuine concern for families with multiples in this study, particularly given that once a placement was available, the family had to pay for it or lose it:

> Even though my husband is unemployed, we have no choice but to pay for the only daycare we found due to the lack of availability of spots for our twins in other day cares. If we passed up these spots, we may not be able to find any available spots when my husband does find a job. (Participant 28)

Beyond paying for an unused placement, mothers also spoke to the impossible and unfair decision that they faced in such situations: should they send one multiple while waiting for a space to open up for the second multiple (or third)? To avoid this, while waiting for spaces, families employed different solutions. Some used unregulated childcare provided by family, friends, or private day homes, and hired nannies; others used the less desirable alternatives of non-subsidized spaces, more expensive programs, and spaces farther from home. Some mothers decided to stay home with their children—temporarily while waiting for childcare or long-term—and a few became childcare providers themselves. These choices had consequences; for example, a mother at home with her three children explained that "I struggled taking care of my oldest and my twins while pregnant with my youngest. I went into labour 3 weeks early" (Participant 29). Clearly, her words evince the strain of childcare on her quality of life.

Mothers who delayed returning to work, often taking unpaid leaves of varying durations, felt they had no other option (e.g., "I had to wait for 2 extra weeks for one of my triplets. I stayed home with him without pay" [Participant 30]). Some became creative in finding ways to pay for childcare or to ensure that children would be placed in quality facilities. For some, these strategies included returning to school (e.g., "I returned to school because that was the only way I could get money for daycare" [Participant 31]). The lack of flexible childcare left many mothers adjusting their work schedules to part time (e.g., "I stayed at home and took flexible part time work" [Participant 32]) or trying different shifts to fit with the childcare available (e.g., "I worked a different shift so coverage was possible" [Participant 33]), while others arranged their work to eliminate the need for childcare (e.g., "I worked nights and we tried babysitters and family for a few hours a day so I could sleep" [Participant 34]). Such strategies also had the latent function of creating marital strain and inducing stress.

Of course, finding flexible childcare that accommodated work schedules was a common difficulty for families (39 percent, *n*=50). Specifically, part-time childcare and childcare suitable to atypical work schedules was near impossible to find (particularly at an affordable rate). The following four participants each highlighted their unique childcare needs and the challenges that such needs created:

Children in care for 4 hours due to medical appointments, then 10 hours next day to make up work time—present daycare charges $10/hour/child whenever over 9 hours of care/day regardless of how many days or hours in care the rest of the week or month. I cannot work shift work as a registered nurse (0700-1915) as daycare is only open 0700-1800. (Participant 35)

My schedule being part time makes my needs change week to week, but I cannot find daycare that can change with it.... This does not help people working part time in lower-income wage jobs who then find it easier to stay home and collect welfare—which I have considered—or fake a separation from my husband so I would be eligible for subsidies. (Participant 36)

I made a major career change because I wanted to pursue both a career and being available for my children. This means we don't need much childcare, where we had been using a full-time nanny up until the girls started school. Availability of childcare that isn't full time and traditional makes it hard to make choices to work differently. It often seems like all or nothing (work full time or stay home). We have had to be very creative and have multiple options for childcare in our bag of tricks to make two careers work out ... the first year back at work with two babies requiring care; we paid a premium because we had twins. (Participant 37)

I travel for work and my husband works out of town as well. I was quoted such high amounts for overnight care that I could not afford to go back to work. They are allowing me to work part time for a few months but then I will have to quit. I make over $80,000 and can't keep my job because I'd be gone too often and would spend 75 percent of my take home on childcare. (Participant 38)

These diverse excerpts reveal the range of families affected by inadequate childcare availability at all levels of socio-economic status. Furthermore, the desperation for some families is clear in these excerpts, as is the strain of finding suitable, available childcare at an affordable price, which was a source of familial stress for many participants.

Moreover, simply finding and managing childcare for evolving schedules requires much time and effort—when clearly families were already over-utilizing their human resources. Common strategies used to find childcare were online resources (30 percent, $n=25$) or relying on word of mouth (29 percent, $n=24$). Respondents reported that they "contacted *all* daycare centres in my area and was put on wait lists" (Participant 39), made "*many* phone calls from online resources" (Participant 40), and did "Research! Research! And more research!" (Participant 41). These excerpts reveal the vast efforts, time, and dedication involved in finding childcare for multiples, which was often a source of stress:

While we were lucky enough to find spots at a daycare we really like, it was very stressful being on waiting lists and knowing that there are very few spaces available in Toronto. Thinking ahead to school years, the kids will have to switch daycares and the issue of finding spaces that offer before and after school care at a location that is convenient to our local school is already creating stress for me. (Participant 42)

Unsurprisingly, it was common for the secondary wage earner to stop working after children are born. In some cases, this parent was away from work temporarily. One respondent indicated "I went on unpaid leave for another year because there was nothing available for 12-month-old children" (Participant 43). Others returned to work part time or with a modified schedule to reduce or eliminate the need for childcare, as previously mentioned, which, of course, affected their career prospects significantly.

SUITABILITY

Finding suitable childcare was a challenge for 59 percent (*n*=76) of surveyed mothers, which included finding high-quality childcare. High-quality childcare in this case was operationalized to include qualified childcare providers in facilities located in close proximity to the mothers' home or work that offer flexible scheduling, who have knowledge of the needs of multiples and can provide support for children with special needs. Even in simply meeting one of the above criteria, such as qualified care providers, mothers expressed distress: "We visited many regulated day homes and wouldn't leave our pets there. There was no way our kids were going there" (Participant 23) or "Our son has special needs and requires his caregivers to have special training" (Participant 45).

Unsurprisingly, mothers overwhelmingly valued government regulation and facility inspection. They appreciated clean, safe spaces with trained staff for both daycare centres and day homes. Specifically, they wanted to see more regulation for in-home childcare and daycare centres in terms of "cleanliness, nutrition, physical activity, developmentally appropriate games and activities, managed by staff with certificates in Early Childhood Education—and paid a good minimum wage" (Participant 46). Some mothers wanted care providers with specific experience and knowledge about multiples; these moms felt multiples were "different than other children" and needed "highly trained individuals ... sensitive to each child's needs" as multiples are not merely "this one and the other one" (Participant 47). This was not a common desire but was put forth by select respondents.

Overall, as posed by Sinha, "Finding the most appropriate child care arrangement can, at times, be challenging. Parents must often balance the need between the overall quality, convenience, availability and cost of child care." Such processes require considerable effort by the mother to identify suitable, affordable, and available childcare and/or to arrange her work schedule to meet the available childcare.

SUGGESTIONS

Addressing the cost of childcare for children was the predominant response from participants when asked about solutions to the challenges they identified as tied to meeting their childcare needs. The general belief was that decreasing service costs while increasing subsidies are needed forms of assistance in paying for childcare. Some mothers further highlighted the needs of families of multiples by suggesting the government provide subsidies based on multiples, total number of children, and net family income. Some urged for the government to become involved in making childcare universally available, while others suggested that families with lower incomes be prioritized to make supplemented financial support depend on income. Furthermore, some respondents felt that subsidies should not penalize families that choose not use childcare (e.g., "[it] would be nice if financial support was available to all families so that families may choose to raise their own children" [Participant 48]), while others held an opposing view, feeling that working parents should be recognized for their contributions to society (e.g., "I think governments need to keep in mind that by working, a number of parents are saving for retirement, which is lessening the burden on government programs in the future" [Participant 24]). Indeed, a number of respondents identified the childcare system in Quebec, where childcare was subsidized at the rate of $7 a day for families (to be increased in 2015), as a model for affordable childcare (Anderssen and Mackrael).

Despite ideas about ways to improve affordability, respondents were quick to identify that such subsidies are useless without sufficient childcare providers available. Thus, on the one hand, mothers wanted more required training for childcare providers, to have small childcare centres in workplaces, and to create "saved" spaces for families with multiple children needing care. Some, on the other hand, took a different approach altogether in advocating for extended leave for families of multiples and for providing support for parents wishing to return to school or to find better employment opportunities. The need for dual parental leave was also highlighted:

> Parents need support so that both parents can be off for the first few months with multiples and receive pay from the government. If I had had my kids separately rather than as twins, I would have received two years of EI [Employment Insurance] pay. However, I only received one. My husband took a three month unpaid leave which cost us between eight and ten thousand dollars. Spouses should be able to use some paid time sometimes so it is fair between people with two singletons and people with twins. (Participant 44)

Of course, some respondents put forth more radical solutions, such as providing free childcare in order for parents to freely return to work; letting moms stay home for two years (one year of maternity leave and one year of a subsidy); hiring nannies for the first month after a child's birth; paying moms to stay home with their children; and subsidizing 80 percent of the cost of childcare.

CONCLUSIONS AND RECOMMENDATIONS

Families with multiples are clearly facing unique challenge as well as intensified versions of the challenges faced by parents of singletons in finding suitable, affordable, and available childcare for their children. Cost and availability are driving concerns in finding care that can lead to lifestyle choices for families of multiples that increase financial stress and caretaking strain. Furthermore, these challenges are made even more difficult with higher order multiples and when their multiple birth children have other siblings.

In response, many mothers report developing individual solutions designed to meet their unique familial needs, including changing work schedules, working fewer hours, not returning to work, using multiple types of childcare, relying on family and friends, and choosing unregulated childcare. While these choices may provide solutions for individual families, they fail to recognize that childcare issues are shared by many families and may require an organized, societal response rather than individual one. Furthermore, these individual choices have social and long-term personal impacts. First, many mothers of multiples are choosing not to return to full-time work after parental leave. (In some cases, mothers are not returning until their children are in school.) This reality negatively affects the long-term employability of the mother, her current and future financial position, and the economy (e.g., more able persons are pushed out of the workforce when the Canadian population is aging quickly and lacks a wide population to draw funds from for pensions and healthcare needs). Second, mothers are continually identifying and coordinating multiple forms of childcare to maintain their employment. In some situations, mothers are also managing employment processes for nannies, or they are volunteering to coordinate parent-run childcare programs, which increases the amount of unpaid work they need to do in order to manage their childcare arrangements. These practices create more occupational and personal stresses and strains being placed on already overworked individuals. Third, family schedules are changing as parents are working opposite shifts or forgoing sleep in order to work and ensure childcare for their children; again all factors that negatively affect social, physical, and psychological health, which in essence, is not sustainable long term.

Another important consideration is that children are being placed in unregulated settings or with providers who are not trained (including family members, nannies and unregulated day homes) that may provide lower-quality care. This reality conflicts with the apparent concern for having qualified childcare providers; it may indicate that this is a secondary concern or that families are simply desperate for care and feel no alternative exists. This situation is particularly common in families with higher order multiples (triplets or more) or twins with one or more siblings, because a nanny is a more cost-effective choice than childcare for three or more children. Nannies are often in Canada as temporary workers leaving their own children to care for Canadian families (Mack-Canty).

While some of these challenges are not unique to families with multiples, the presence of two or more children of the same age increases the cost of childcare and decreases the availability. There are currently no specific supports for these families, beyond sibling discounts, that provide limited financial benefits to families. Furthermore, the lack of available childcare for infants (i.e., two or more available placements in one centre for twins, triplets or quadruplets) creates a new source of strain for parents who require care for multiple children. This situation can lead to stressful decision-making or unnecessary expenditures such as paying for placement while waiting for an additional spot to open up for the sibling.

In light of these concerns, there is a need to increase available supports for families with multiples to ensure that they have access to affordable and regulated childcare that meets these families' unique needs (International Council of Multiple Birth Organisations and International Society for Twin Studies). Dual parental leave to support families to care for their infants, policies to make placing multiples in childcare facilities easier, and subsidies based on number of children and family income—all may assist with overcoming some of the challenges related to finding childcare for multiples; however, it does not solve the current dilemma. Furthermore, it must be recognized that as long as there are not enough spots available for children in diverse childcare settings, this will divide families, as persons are basically competing for needed services. Such realities create additional stress for mothers and burden families. Quality childcare allows children to benefit from interactions with their peers, improves school readiness, and provides numeracy and language skills (OECD). The lack of available regulated childcare for all multiple birth children can stratify children—including by socio-economic status—before they start school. With higher rates of some developmental delays, including speech delays in multiples (MBC, "Multiple Births Facts and Figures"; MBC, "Speech and Language Development"), the negative outcomes of not providing high quality childcare can be magnified.

Like all Canadian mothers, mothers of multiples tried to accommodate to their situations by locating and using available the childcare options in their community —that is hoped to be suitable and affordable. Given the limited childcare options, mothers are often adjusting their schedules, changing or leaving their jobs, and bringing together a myriad of multiple sources of childcare to meet the needs of their family. They clearly see childcare as an individual issue rather than a social concern. Overall, there is little concern for the greater social implications tied to the limited childcare options for mothers of multiples. Consequently, these women, who often have many years of schooling and experience invested in their careers, are *choosing*—they genuinely lack any alterative options (thus it is not a choice per se)—to change careers or stay home because of the lack of available childcare. Policy decisions, such as failing to offer parental leave for each child in a multiple birth family, further shift the burden of responsibility to individual families, resulting in negative long terms effects on the family's well-being.

NOTES

[1]Erroneous responses (e.g., a respondent indicating she pays $250/ hour for childcare) were removed.

[2]The regional distribution of participants is largely English speaking and reflects, to some degree, the geographic location of MBC chapters (most are located in Ontario at the time of the survey, with one chapter in Alberta and one in British Columbia).

WORKS CITED

Amoroso, Julie. "From Women to Children: Reframing Child Care in Canada." *Queen's Policy Review* 1.1 (2010): 29-46. Web. 14 January 2015.

Anderssen, Erin, and Kim Mackrael. "Better Daycare for $7/Day: One Province's Solution for Canada." *Globe and Mail*, 18 October 2013. Web. 14 January 2015.

Best Start: Ontario's Maternal, Newborn and Early Child Development Resource Centre with Multiple Births Canada. "Low Birth Weight & Preterm Multiple Births: A Canadian Profile." MBC, 2005. Web. 14 January 2015.

Davis, Elizabeth, and Rachel Connelly. "The Influence of Local Price and Availability on Parents' Choice of Childcare." *Population Research and Policy Review* 24.4 (2005): 301-334. Web. 14 January 2015.

Fisher, Jane. "Psychological and Social Implications of Multiple Gestation and Birth." *Australian and New Zealand Journal of Obstetrics and Gynaecology* 46. Supplement S1 (2006): S34–S37. Web. 14 January 2015.

Glazebrook, Cris, Charlotte Sheard, Sara Cox, Margaret Oates, and George Ndukwe. "Parenting Stress in First-time Mothers of Twins and Triplets Conceived After In Vitro Fertilization." *Fertility and Sterility* 8.3 (2004): 505-511. Web. 14 January 2015.

Hankins, Gary, and George Saade. "Factors Influencing Twins and Zygosity." *Paediatric & Perinatal Epidemiology* 19. Supplement S1 (2005): 8-9. Web. 14 January 2015.

Holland, Mary. "Funding and Framing Families: An Analysis of the Discursive Foundations of Family Allowance and the Universal Child Care Benefit." *Journal of the Motherhood Initiative for Research & Community* 3.1 (2012): 39-52. Web. 14 January 2015.

International Council of Multiple Birth Organisations and International Society for Twin Studies. "Declaration of Rights and Statement of Needs of Twins and Higher Order Multiples." MBC, 2007. Web. 14 January 2015.

Immervoll, Herwig and David Barber. "Can Parents Afford to Work? Childcare Costs, Tax-Benefit Policies and Work Incentives." *IZA Discussion Papers, Forschungsinstitut zur Zukunft der Arbeit* No. 1932 (2006). Web. 14 January 2015.

Mack-Canty, Colleen. "The Global Restructuring of Care: The Third World Nanny Phenomenon." *Journal of the Association for Research on Mothering* 10.1 (2008): 107-118. Web. 14 January 2015.

McKinley, Renée. *Childcare by Choice or by Default? Examining the Experiences of Unregulated Home-based Childcare for Women in Paid Work and Training.* Diss. *Brock University Digital*

Repository. Brock University, 2015. Web. 14 January 2015.

McKay, Stephen. "The Effects of Twins and Multiple Births on Families and Their Living Standards." Twins and Multiple Births Association (TAMBA), 2010. Web. 14 January 2015.

Multiple Births Canada (MBC). "Multiple Births Facts and Figures." MBC, 2011. Web. 14 January 2015.

Multiple Births Canada (MBC). "Supreme Court of Canada Decision. Parental Leave Benefits Will Not Be Argued in Court." MBC, 2013. Web. 14 January 2015.

Multiple Births Canada (MBC). "Speech and Language Development for Children of Multiple Birth." *Multiple Births Canada*. Multiple Births Canada, 2014. Web. 14 January 2015.

Nguyen, Linda. "Ontario City Has Least Affordable Child Care in Canada, Study Says." *theglobeandmail.com*. The Globe and Mail, 10 Nov 2014. Web. 14 January 2015.

Noakes, Susan. "Child-Care Affordability Varies Widely Across Canada: Brampton, Ont., Least Affordable, Gatineau, Que., the Most Affordable." Canadian Broadcasting Corporation, 10 Nov 2014. Web. 14 January 2015.

Organization for Economic Co-Operation and Development (OECD). "Starting Strong II: Early Childhood Education and Care—Final Report of the Thematic Review of Early Childhood Education and Care."OECD, 2006. Web. 14 January 2015.

Prentice, Susan. "Childcare, Co-production, and the Third Sector in Canada." *Public Management Review* 8.4 (2006): 521-536. Web. 14 January 2015.

Prentice, Susan. "Less Access, Worse Quality: New Evidence about Poor Children and Regulated Child Care in Canada." *Journal of Children and Poverty* 13.1 (2007): 57-73. Web. 14 January 2015.

Robin, Monique, Denis Corroyer, and Irene Casati. "Childcare Patterns of Mothers of Twins during the First Year." *Journal of Child Psychology and Psychiatry* 37.4 (1996): 453-460. Web. 14 January 2015.

Sinha, Marie. "Analytical Paper: Child Care in Canada." *Statistics Canada*. Government of Canada, 2014. Web. 14 January 2015.

Visual Interlude III

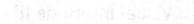

9.
The Art of Twinning

VICTORIA TEAM

ARTIST'S STATEMENT

I am an Australian women's health researcher. Currently, I am working on the collaborative project *Contraceptive Technologies and Reproductive Choice Among Immigrant and Refugee Women in Australia* run by the School of Social Sciences at Monash University. I was born in eastern Ukraine, where I was also trained as a general practitioner. I then practised in Ethiopia for over ten years. I undertook a six-month obstetrics and gynecology internship at St. Paul's Hospital, Addis Ababa, where I worked both at the antenatal clinic and maternity ward as scheduled.

When I am deeply touched by events, clinical cases, patient stories, experiences of research participants, and my own experiences, I feel a need to communicate these feelings and experiences to others, either through writing or pot painting. I am not a professional painter; pot painting is my hobby. I purchase terracotta and clay pots in the opportunity shops and in second-hand markets. I usually use black oil paint mixed with linseed oil and create black-and-red images, similar with the images on Ancient Greek vases. I feel that I might have inherited some talents from my Greek grandmother, Maria Kharakhursakh, who was a talented painter. Although she was semi-literate, she was invited to work at one of the Soviet animation studios. I further learned some aspects of sketching, drawing and oil painting from my stepfather, Vladimir Korostil, who was a professional painter.

The *Twinning in Africa* urn is dedicated to one of my patients, an Ethiopian woman who had two twin sets and came to the clinic that I worked in for an antenatal check-up. She suspected she had a twin pregnancy, and this was later confirmed by the ultrasound findings. The central image of the urn depicts an African woman, pregnant with twins, breastfeeding twin infants while surrounded by her twin toddlers, who are seeking attention. The design around the neck of the urn represents multiple twin sets.

In my second artwork, *Twin Pregnancy: The Body, Mind, and Soul* urn, I attempt to present twin pregnancy, applying a holistic perspective. With twin pregnancy, in addition to body changes and feelings—including heaviness, pressure, and tiredness related to carrying a large belly—women's minds and souls are also affected. Women may worry about the outcome of the pregnancy and potential complications; they might also think about their ability to breastfeed and care for twins. The *Twin Pregnancy: The Body, Mind, and Soul* image can be seen in more than one way: as a face, as a heart, and as a uterus, where the face represents the mind, heart represents the soul, and uterus represents the body. Spiral shapes on the top may represent hair if you see the image as a woman's face; they may represent major heart vessels if you see this image as a heart or be seen as *chorionic villi* if you see this image as a uterus. Fetus hands could be viewed as maternal eyes or also as a heart valve; lips on this image could also be viewed as the opening of the womb.

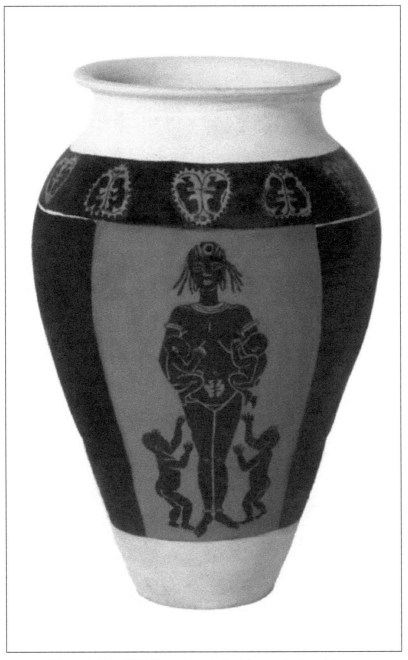

Twinning in Africa. 2015. Linseed-based oil paint on a red coloured clay urn,
15 ¾ X 8^{17}/$_{64}$ X 8^{17}/$_{64}$ inches. Image by: Robert Lean

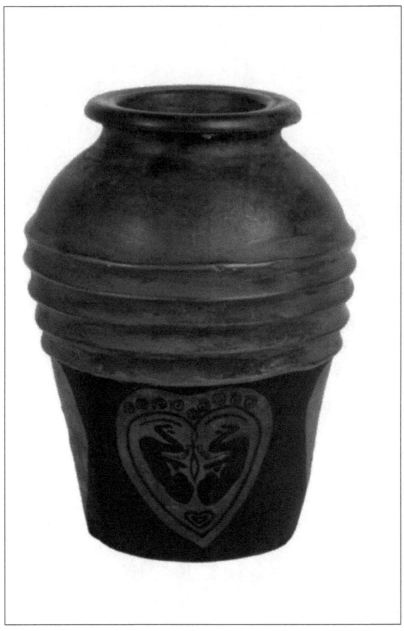

Twin pregnancy: The Body, Mind, and Soul. 2015. Linseed-based oil paint on a mahogany coloured clay urn, 15 ¾ X 8$^{17}/_{64}$ X 8$^{17}/_{64}$ inches. Image by: Robert Lean

10.
Queer Parenting and the Revelation of Twins

LESLIE ROBERTSON AND KATHRYN TREVENEN

W E START THIS ESSAY with a quote from a blog titled "Why Are There Always Rainbow Flags at Pro-Abortion Rallies?" in which we were referenced after attending a protest to the March for Life on Parliament Hill in 2011, during the first month we were dating. The author wrote, "it's no coincidence that at this year's National March for Life in Ottawa, the award for most –'ingenious' sign went to a pair of lesbians, who were ostentatiously showing 'affection' holding two different card-board cut-outs, one that said 'I LOVE SEX' and the other, 'I HATE LIFE'" (Golob). The anti-abortion protest happens every year, and as a part of the counter-protest, we spray-painted these irreverent signs. As many of our fellow counter-protestors pointed out, these were not particularly helpful or nuanced signs (indeed!), but we got a lot of laughs, and the signs captured our weariness with trying to engage thoughtfully with an anti-abortion movement that seemed so rigid and woman hating. Our signs and our tongue-in-cheek message inspired anti-abortion activist Alissa Golob to write the above blog post for *Life Site News*, a website, about the close connections between "homosexuality" and "pro-abortion" positions. Lining up the "sterility," "individualism," and un(re)productiveness of homosexuality against the supposed fertility, unity and (re)productiveness of heterosexuality, Golob argues that it makes sense for "the homosexual" to be in favour of abortion because homosexuality corresponds with the rejection and destruction of life. She writes that, "homosexuality uses sex as an instrument for self-gratifying pleasure, and cannot physically be used in the unitive and procreative way it was intended." Reading the blog, we laughed, shook our heads at the intersecting homophobia and heteronormativity in the piece and felt very queer.

Two years later, those two abortion-loving, life-hating, self-gratifying queers were pregnant with twins.

This essay pursues questions and concerns coming out of our reflections on our queer family and baby making and out of the seeming contradiction between the two different moments in our life outlined above. In the first moment, our queerness seemed obvious. We were performing visible queerness with in-your-face feminist protest, ostentatious affection, a community of people around us, and the right-wing attacked us. In the second moment, we had (mostly) held our tongues and tolerated heteronormative processes while visiting fertility clinics. Were we still queer? Can people with twins *be* queer?

Our contribution asks and answers this question in several ways. As a same-sex couple who ultimately used in vitro fertilization (IVF) to conceive our babies with an egg donating mama (Leslie) and a gestating mama (Kathryn), we reflect in the first section of the essay on our experience of queer reproduction and contrast the intensely communal, queer, and playful nature of our original attempts to get pregnant with the surprisingly heteronormative and "traditional" environment of the fertility clinic and IVF. In this section, we examine the privilege that is integral to how we were able to conceive our babies and also reflect on the disciplining effects of the medicalization of reproduction and our attempts at resistance. We will use this section of the essay to both interrogate the inaccessibility of many fertility treatments in Canada (especially ones that require the extra expense of donor sperm and eggs) and to celebrate the ways that chosen family and friends supported us through the conception process. Central to this first section is a consideration of homonormativity, queer family, and our own questions about what was "queer" about this baby-making process.

The second section of the essay asks if there is something *particularly* queer about multiples, in our case twins. We reflect on the ways that having two babies necessarily and joyfully queered our experience of early parenting—from being two breastfeeding women, to an unanticipated level of involvement from friends and family, and to reflections about gender norms and the complexity of raising a boy and a girl at the same time. We hope that by posing these questions, we can nuance the complex and fraught personal politics of engaging with the fertility industry, having "IVF twins," and exploring our role as queer parents in the context of the challenge of raising multiple babies.

Throughout the paper, we follow Nikki Sullivan in understanding the concept of "queer" to be centrally concerned with disrupting normative and "normalising ways of knowing and of being" (vi). To "queer" thus means "to make strange, to frustrate, to counteract, to delegitimize, to camp up—heteronormative knowledges and institutions, and the subjectivities and socialities that are (in)formed by them and that (in)form them" (vi). Queerness isn't reducible to sexual practice, identity, or orientation. A consideration of what it means to be queer parents, therefore, and to "parent queerly" is part of the conversation that many queer parents are having—especially as more LGBTQ folks gain access to, and resources for, parenting. As Rachel Epstein argues in *Who's Your Daddy? And Other Writings on Queer Parenting*, parenting queerly might not be simply or primarily about identity (where parents identify as LGBTQ) but instead about "something more intentional and/or radical" (27). Epstein explores what it would mean to see queer parenting as being about non-normative parenting that challenges norms around things such as family structure and/or composition, domestic space, "family time," and reproduction (323). Epstein highlights the challenges of "resisting normal" in our orientations to things such as parenting, family structure, or gender—both because there is something profoundly heteronormative about reproduction in North American culture, and because many queer parents want to protect their children from rejection or marginalization by being as "normal" as possible.

For Epstein, queerness and being a "queer parent" are not stable or consistent processes or subject positions. As queer theoretical considerations of homonormativity and homonationalism reveal, some queer subjects and families are actively supported and cultivated, while others are targeted for increased marginalization and exclusion. In *The Twilight of Equality*, queer theorist Lisa Duggan examines what she calls the "new homonormativity," a sexual politics that "does not contest dominant heteronormative assumptions and institutions, but upholds and sustains them, while promising the possibility of a demobilized gay constituency and a privatized, depoliticized gay culture anchored in domesticity and consumption" (Duggan 50). Campaigns for equal marriage, the gentrification of gay neighbourhoods/the gay village, and representations of the growing numbers of "good," "productive" queers who want children all participate in this new homonormativity.

In *Terrorist Assemblages: Homonationalism in Queer Times*, Jasbir Puar extends Duggan's critique of neoliberal homonormativity to examine how homonormativity works not simply to distinguish between the "good gays" and the bad queers," but also how queerness "as a process of racialization informs the very distinctions between life and death, wealth and poverty, health and illness, living and dying" (xi). Puar highlights how the temporary inclusion of certain queer subjects supports different national and imperial projects, and how extending limited equality rights to some homonational citizens masks the ongoing queering of racialized, "terrorist" populations who are marked for death. The fertility industry and the politics of queer reproduction throw many of these necropolitical power relations into stark relief.

Throughout this paper, we argue that these homonational and homonormative relations of power characterize our considerations and experiences of queer baby making and queer parenting. We argue that twins queered our baby-making and baby-raising experiences and strategies in interesting and unexpected ways, opening our lives up and disturbing norms of parenting, even as we were increasingly aware of our homonormativity and our privilege. At times, it was our very homonational privilege that allowed us to queer processes of reproduction and family structure; at other times, it was the fact that we had twins that queered our orientation to parenting and community. Ultimately, we argue that, for us, twins themselves create a queer excess to the norm and that they queered our lives, family structures, and relationships in important ways—from how we understand gender construction, to whom we identify as playing parental roles.

QUEER CONCEPTION?
MULTIPLE MOTHERS CONCEIVE MULTIPLES

We had a lot of fun trying to conceive our babies, and not because it involved a lot of sex with each other. Like a growing number of parents, our twins were ultimately conceived by way of in vitro fertilization. However, we didn't start out doing IVF, and the journey that got us there was a community project in many different ways. From finding sperm, to multiple do-it-yourself (DIY) rounds of what we called "inspermination," and to dealing with the challenges of the fertility industry, our queer family was actively involved in the process.

In the collection *And Baby Makes More: Known Donors Queer Parents and Our Unexpected Families*, editors Chloë Brushwood Rose and Susan Goldberg argue that procreating in the queer community often involves "more people, more intimacy, more negotiating, processing and imagining than a typical hetero couple" (8). The collection tells many different stories of the ways in which friendships and alternative families form to create babies, and how babies then change those friendships and families. As Brushwood Rose and Goldberg maintain, "love makes a family but also courage, patience, flexibility, generosity, and a sort of inclusion that can accommodate the unknown ways in which people may or may not come together to make a family" (8). Our experience reflects these themes and these complex, unexpected, and joyful intimacies and negotiations.

One of the first tasks we looked to our queer family for help with was finding sperm. Initially, we shopped online via an international sperm bank, and we had a sperm search committee comprised of Aunties Vanessa and Sara, who were tasked with choosing "Mr. Right." We met over a weekday evening (Sara) and a fall weekend at a friend's cottage (Vanessa) armed with good food, wine, copies of a long list of perspective donor profiles, file folders, and a rainbow of highlighters and sharpies. The committee turned the long list into a short list and the short list into a vote that narrowed it down to one donor. At this point in the process, the plan was to use a fertility clinic to perform IUI (intrauterine insemination) to try to get Kathryn pregnant. As Kathryn was thirty-nine by that point, the doctor at the fertility clinic highlighted the need to move quickly.

We tried four rounds of IUI at the fertility clinic, and although the nurses were extremely friendly, professional, and helpful, we generally did not find the doctors, the forms, or the environment to be particularly welcoming or sensitive to queer lives, experiences, and family styles. Combined with a growing sense that anonymous sperm didn't feel right for us and discomfort with the fertility clinic, we began to think about asking a friend to give us sperm so that we could try to get pregnant "the old fashioned way"—with a syringe, a bottle of wine, and a bunch of our closest friends. The benefits of using a friend's sperm seemed compelling to us. Using friendly sperm would provide us with medical information and provide our potential future children with answers about the humans involved in their creation. As many straight people do, we wanted to make our babies with people we love and respect. Many folks prefer to use anonymous sperm to avoid the possibility of legal or emotional complications and to protect the precarious legal status of the "second parent." This makes absolute sense to us, but in our case, we decided that the risks and complexities of known sperm were worth it.

It did not take long to broker a sperm deal within our community. We asked a good friend of ours, David, and he accepted after we established that all three of us agreed on his role as a friend to a future baby, but not a parent (a role that he would have played regardless of the sperm used to conceive the babies). When we sat down to discuss the logistics of this deal, and our needs and expectations, David compared giving us sperm to us loaning him a cottage for a week. If he had something we needed or wanted, he would be happy to give it to us, just as we would happily give him something he needed or wanted. We also agreed that we didn't want a legal contract to sanction our agreement. Since we were all committed to challenging state policing of borders, relationships, and bodies, we felt that we didn't need the legal system regulating our relationships with future children. We also opted out of doing a third party adoption, whereby Leslie would have adopted the children from David. These types of adoptions are still a common way for non-gestational moms to obtain legal status as a parent when their children are conceived by way of known donors, but we were lucky enough to feel confident that David would never challenge our right to parent our children.

In making this decision, we recognized the generations of queer families that came before us who enabled us to reject these onerous, expensive, and offensive legal formalities. Decades of hard-fought custody battles by lesbian mothers now allow us to feel confident in our status as parents, even while consciously choosing not to legally sanction our families in what remains a very uncertain legal landscape in Ontario for children conceived using known donors.[1] Here we also feel the impact of our considerable homonormative/ homonational privilege. As cis, white, financially privileged women who have access to legal and community support, and who have stable status as Canadian citizens, we do not expect a high level of surveillance of our family, or police or state intervention in our family or home. In many ways, our ability to cultivate our "queer/non-normative" orientation to baby making (known donor, no legal agreement) is a direct result of our privilege and our protected status.

After the uncomfortable environment of the fertility clinic, trying to get pregnant at home with friends felt both optimistic and joyful. Over several attempts at DIY insemination—aka insperminization—we developed a ritual that we looked forward to. We spent long evenings cooking, drinking wine, dancing and laughing—all around the exchange of an appreciated (and slightly warm) syringe of semen. We also got creative around ovulation time, converging in different cities, hotels, bathrooms, other people's beds, and at other professional and life events. In addition to being a fun excuse to hang out with people we love, this celebration of the insperminization process deeply challenged a lot of the negative messages our culture produces around reproduction and "infertility." While we felt vulnerable and abnormal in the environment of the fertility clinic, we felt loved and supported eating and drinking with our people. Our queer family sustained and inspired us—especially as months passed and Kathryn didn't get pregnant.

Like other procreating teams, our anxiety about being able to conceive grew with the unsuccessful insperminization attempts. Eventually, our fun group project led to a more stressful, expensive, and anxiety-producing stage when it was recommended that we try IVF. Inspermination went from a monthly ritual gathering we celebrated with friends to being a series of medicalized procedures and legal formalities as dictated by the fertility clinic that we had to once again engage with. We agreed to try IVF on the recommendation of fertility doctors, considering that Kathryn, who was trying to conceive, was now over forty years old. We decided to use Leslie's eggs (she is seven years younger) to increase our chances of getting pregnant. At the time, we weren't aware of the characterization of this process as "Lesbian IVF"—a process in which one woman donates eggs and one woman carries. As Epstein explains, although queer parents often argue that love, and not biology, matters, "to say that biology doesn't matter in the creation of our families does not fully capture our reproductive desires and motivations, nor does it reflect what we actually do reproductively" (91). Epstein further argues that the re-appropriation of IVF for queer conception, "underscores the hegemonic, heteronormative cultural presumption that only mutual biological contributions result in a 'real' co-creation" (86).

We feel a complicated ambivalence towards this argument. On the one hand, we both felt that any children we had (by any means) would be our "real" children, regardless of whose genetics were involved. We pursued donor egg IVF because IVF is very expensive and we were told that "younger" eggs gave us a better chance of conceiving. The decision was practical and financial. But on the other hand we clearly both did have complex attachments to biological aspects of the process. Kathryn wanted (if possible) to experience pregnancy, and Leslie now gets a kick out of the fact that the twins look like her and enjoys that she is perceived publicly as their "real mother" and not assumed to be less legitimately a parent.

These attachments and ambivalences arose in part as a result of our engagement with the fertility clinic that we used. Our unique situation of partner egg donation and using sperm from a known donor challenged the clinic policy and operation and was a constant reminder of how we were at the mercy of a largely heteronormative industry. It became clear to us that the clinic's operational starting point was straight couples with fertility challenges and that the more we didn't fit into that framework, the less equipped they were to deal with us. We were given literature about coping with infertility and a pamphlet on how and if to tell children they were conceived using donor sperm. We were also mandated to get cleared by a psychologist as individuals who were donating and receiving genetic material, and were made to sign irrelevant and offensive legal waivers. The forms the clinic made us sign were clearly designed for a woman in a straight couple receiving sperm from an anonymous donor and eggs from another woman in a straight couple. The very first line of the egg donor waiver clarified that an egg donor has no legal parental rights to the potential child. The document also had the egg donor's "husband or spouse" waiving his parental claims to the child and the donor agreeing to abstain from sex with her (male) spouse while undergoing the treatment for egg donation. The message we took from these forms was that these processes were not for us.

Our biggest challenge with fertility laws and procedures in Canada was the insistence on treating our friend's semen as an unknown and potentially threatening substance. Canadian law requires physicians to quarantine sperm for six months before administering it, unless it is from a "spouse" or a "sexual partner."[2] The rationale for this quarantine is that it allows doctors to test the sperm to prevent the transmission of sexually transmitted infections, notably HIV. The requirement for quarantine limits the liability of the doctor or institution with regard to a patient who hasn't otherwise previously assumed the risk associated with having "sex" with the donor. Being aware of the law regulating physician-administered sperm, we clearly communicated that we considered our donor to be Kathryn's sexual partner. We also explained that we had used his semen numerous times—thus assuming the same risks as having unprotected sex. At this explanation, our doctor asked Kathryn to specify what type of sex she had and whether she had had intercourse with him. When we then asked the doctor whether he asked straight couples to specify what type of sex they had, he responded that of course he didn't. Since Kathryn conceded to not having intercourse with our sperm donor, the clinic refused to perform IVF with our sperm without first quarantining it for six months. This requirement resulted in the sperm having to go to a different clinic in a different city to be tested, stored, and shipped. This process not only cost thousands of dollars, it also delayed our ability to do IVF by seven months, which, by our doctor's own account, was not insignificant in terms of fertility for women our ages.

Ultimately, we were able to pursue IVF, and Kathryn became pregnant with twins. Our financial privilege allowed us access to reproductive technology and resources that many people cannot access. We were privileged to live in a city with a fertility clinic (despite its limitations), to have professional flexibility that allowed us to take time off to undergo the treatments and procedures, and to have drug plan that covered the cost of the drugs. Here again, our homonormative privilege was also clear amid the challenges. Although the forms at the clinic didn't include us, we also weren't assumed to be dangerous or threatening in our desire to reproduce, and the sense of entitlement that we felt to services reflects the entitlement that comes along with white supremacy—the assumption that white lives are worth sustaining and producing. At every stage in the process, we felt the impact of our race and class privilege and saw the precarity with which reproductive justice and care is extended to marginalized people.

We were also very fortunate to have amazing networks of support from our communities and families that not only got us through the making babies stage but continued to help keep us alive and thriving postpartum and beyond. It was this support that sustained us emotionally throughout our interactions with the fertility clinic—interactions that we had little ability to change or combat. If we wanted access to the technology and expertise necessary for IVF, we had to agree to their policies and restrictions. Despite the normalizing and disciplining impacts of engaging with "the fertility industry," it was the support and enthusiasm from our community that sustained many of our reproductive efforts.

MULTIPLES AND THE QUEER FAMILY MODEL

As a same-sex couple, we needed to look beyond our partnership in order to conceive, and as parents of multiples we once again came to rely on the generosity of our community and on forming new family relations and structures to survive the challenges of simultaneously caring for two new premature babies. Our families of origin and our large network of chosen family have always been a central part of our lives, and bringing two babies into the fold has strengthened and intensified these relationships in surprising and inspiring ways. We have been dependent on our communities for emotional and logistical support since the babies have been born, and the twins have blown open our family unit in unanticipated ways. Having twins has highlighted our aspirations for queer family models and queer parenting in four key ways. The first is in relation to our extended queer family networks—networks that happily include our families of origin as well.

One of the very first significant postpartum challenges we were faced with was taking home two premature infants while Kathryn was recovering from a C-section. Evidence of the work our friends and family had done met us upon our arrival from the hospital: the house had been cleaned up from the party we had the night before Kathryn went into labour, our driveway and front steps had been shoveled after the first storm of the season, car seats had been installed, and the welcome home banner had been hung. Since Kathryn's mobility was severely restricted post-surgery, we also had a lineup of friends sign up to stay with us for the first weeks we were home.

Those first few weeks and months remain some of the most intense, frightening, and amazing of our lives. Most new parents can relate to the haze of feeding, diapers, crying, and sleeplessness, when the days and nights are interchangeable, and your existence is entirely devoted to sustaining tiny beings. We survived this time thanks to our "famjam" (our queer family, families of origin, and beloved friends) who, among other things, pitched in by bringing us meals for months (thank you food train!!), holding babies, watching babies, changing diapers, passing on baby clothes and baby gear, answering our calls, cleaning our house, fixing our house, delivering groceries, and keeping us company. To say that we had support is an understatement and in writing this account, we are once again overwhelmed and humbled by the love that our families and friends have shared with us. We would wish that all twin parents had this network.

This extended network of support is one of the central pillars of our queer parenting. And in many ways, we argue that twins *are* queer in the ways they challenge the norms of parenting, especially parenting newborns. While many friends and parenting books and blogs encourage new parents to cocoon and take time to themselves when a baby is first born, having two babies and a C-section meant that we were forced to accept help immediately and intensively. This forced openness to our community was uncomfortable at times (both of us had trouble asking for, and accepting, help before the babies were born), but as our friend Fred expressed to us early after the babies were born, being totally overwhelmed also led us to welcome people into our lives in more intimate ways than we might have otherwise done. We were forced to share our babies and share our struggles and this in turn brought many people closer to all four of us.

Having twins has without question intensified our relationships with our friends and family. Both sets of grandparents have travelled long distances to camp out on our pullout couch and act as live-in caregivers for weeks at a time. We have also developed a de facto open door policy for our home. We have a scheduled rotation of chosen family members who come by to help outnumber the babies at key points in the day and folks will often spontaneously stop by for a cuddle, a meal or for bath time—keeping a mama company and/or a baby occupied. As a result, the babies have already become attached to some of their regular visitors, and they often wave at the door and start walking toward it before we've even realized that someone has knocked. We have also discovered our place in the subcultures of parents of multiples, queer parents, and queer parents of multiples—the last one being a pretty small niche. We are very lucky to live among many other non-traditional families and queer parents and to participate in organizations like the Ten Oaks Project that both facilitates summer camps for "queerspawn" (children of queer parents and families) and LGBTQ youth and puts on events to bring these families together all year long.

A second pillar of our experience of the "queerness" of twins is the fact that we both have been able to breastfeed our babies (something that we might not have attempted with only one baby). As the non-gestational mother, Leslie followed a protocol designed for mothers with low milk supply, trans-feminine mothers, or adoptive mothers, which allowed her to breastfeed, despite having never been pregnant. This double breastfeeding situation was in many ways ideal for twin parenting since it took some of the pressure off of each of us. Between the two of us, someone was always attached to a breast pump or a baby. It became such a regular occurrence for our friends and family (and neighbours) to see our breasts that we began to do away with putting on shirts. A layer of intimacy that we had not anticipated experiencing evolved out of this process. Having the focus be on such an outwardly feminine part of her body was particularly challenging for Leslie as someone who identifies as masculine of centre. Ultimately, however, breastfeeding resulted in Leslie developing a new appreciation for her body and was an unexpected twist in her experience of her genderqueer and gender non-conforming identity. Double breastfeeding also marked us as queer when we were in public in a way that felt both vulnerable and affirming.

A third and perhaps most surprising aspect of our queer parenting has come from the evolving inclusion of a third parental figure. Uncle Paul, Kathryn's ex-partner of fifteen years and closest friend, was involved from the beginning of the pregnancy, cheering us on as we got ready to have twins. Once the babies were born, and again in part because of our intense needs in the early months, Paul became an almost daily member of our household. From the beginning, he was our logistical rock, picking up supplies, groceries, prescriptions, and red wine as needed. He was also immediately a direct caregiver for the babies—holding sleeping babies on his chest or taking a baby for a walk in the carrier to give breathing room to the other. We are also indebted to feminist and queer reflections on domestic labour that guide us in dividing tasks between more than two people—especially in the 4:00 p.m. to 7:00 p.m. window when everyone is tired and in need of an extra pair of hands. Paul doesn't just do the "fun" stuff, he changes diapers, holds crying babies as well as laughing ones, and cheerfully gives up his Saturday night date plans to stay home with the kids while we go out.

Paul's daily participation has taken us all by surprise—we didn't plan for it and as the babies have become more and more attached to him (at one point, our daughter pulled up his shirt and seemed to be considering whether or not he was part of the milk bar, and our son now has a particular "smug" look that he only has when Uncle Paul is carrying him around), we have been considering him as a hybrid of uncle and parent. His commitment to the babies and his love for them (and theirs for him) have caused us all to think about the ways the three of us are now accountable to the babies and responsible for this relationship and its continuance.

Many people who see Paul with the babies assume that he is the sperm donor and that the bond they have is biologically driven. This is an interesting assumption that points to the ways in which biological parents are assumed to be the norm—even in a society where many children are raised by adoptive, step, or chosen parents. Paul's relationship with the twins has challenged the supremacy of this biological bond and has also made us think about future possibilities for the relationships the three of them will have. Our daughter has just learned to say Paul's name (her first name other than "mama"), but we are curious to see what else he will be called over the course of their relationship. Parenting blogs, forums, publications, and representations in popular culture are increasingly recognizing the presence of polyamorous parenting groups, and we are also curious about how our "platonic polyamorous" assemblage will be regarded once the twins enter institutions such as the school system. Regardless of what the future will bring for these relationships, we feel very lucky to have had twins that could help guide us through new forms of attachment, family building, and parenting.

The final aspect of queer parenting that the twins have highlighted concerns thinking about gender norms. As feminists who think a lot about gender construction, cisnormativity, transphobia-transmisogyny, and the myriad ways that our society polices children and parents around gender, parenting children who were designated boy and girl at birth has been challenging and revealing. We have experienced the pressure and anxiety that comes with trying to equip our children for a harsh and gendered world, while, at the same time, we have tried to leave their options for gender expression and identity as open as possible. Many of the superficial markers of gender are easy to avoid at an early stage—as infants the twins shared clothes and toys that rarely seemed explicitly marked as for "girls" or for "boys." As the babies have gotten older, however, we've seen that our default to "gender neutral" is heavily skewed toward traditionally masculine toys, clothes, or colours. Dressing our kids in blues, greens, and blacks seems much easier, less controversial, and less provocative than dressing them both in pinks or in dresses, skirts, or clothes that are marked as feminine. Our comfort level with dressing our son in dresses and in pink is much lower, even though he is beautiful in those colours and styles. This experience has pointed to the deep devaluing and hatred of femininity in our culture that Julia Serano explores in *Whipping Girl: A Transsexual Woman on Sexism and the Scapegoating of Femininity* and to the tensions that we feel when we seem to dress our children in ways that "make a statement." We often feel like feminist "killjoys," as Sara Ahmed calls them, because we can't just happily orient ourselves "properly" to gender norms. We've stopped correcting strangers when they comment on our two boys or girls as it's exhausting to always be justifying why our kids are both dressed in blue or wearing frilly clothes, or how it is that a boy can also drink out of a pink sippie cup or wear purple hand-me-down rubber boots.

We are continually in a process of trying to figure out how to introduce our children to a range of options for their gender presentation and identity at the earliest possible stage while also respecting their right to align with gender norms if they choose. For Kathryn, who identifies as a queer femme, it is increasingly important to both model and cultivate an appreciation of femininity for both babies. Leslie has similarly reflected on her gender expression, and on her experience as a masculine-of-centre, genderqueer person. Having a boy and a girl to raise *at the same time* has accentuated the impact of gender norms and policing in a way that seems particular to raising multiples. We feel grateful and indebted to the many gender non-conforming, trans and gender fluid people we know who continue to teach us about unlearning violent gender norms and about new paths to freedom and fulfillment.

Throughout this paper, and the several years we have spent trying to get pregnant, expecting twins and now raising twins, the complexities of our queer lives and of parenting twins have challenged and excited us. Although the process of becoming pregnant with twins highlighted some of the hardest edges of the heteronormative fertility industry and the racist necropolitics underlying queer reproduction and reproductive (in)justice, the experience of having twins has made our understanding of queer family and community more robust and more joyful. Our paper ends with a mixed answer to the questions we started with: can we be queer and have twins? Yes—in fact, having twins has highlighted many things about contemporary queer politics for us: the impact of financial privilege and homonormativity on who has access to reproduction and in what ways; the importance of building community as a response to heteronormative models of the nuclear family; and the sense of openness and possibility that models of queer parenting create for us around family structure, gender norms, and parental roles. Is there something queer about twins themselves? Yes—for us, having twins has both forced and invited us to think more broadly and less normatively about our role as parents and about the community we want our children to have around them. We hope that this openness and excitement will continue to grow as they do.

NOTES

[1] For a more detailed discussion of how different Canadian provinces legislate intentional non-traditional lesbian-lead families see Kelly. See also Miriam Smith and Brenda Cossman for broader discussions of political and legal regulation of queer subjects in Canada.
[2] Processing and Distribution of Semen for Assisted Conception Regulations, S.O.R./2000-410, s.2.

WORKS CITED

Ahmed, Sara. *The Promise of Happiness*. Durham: Duke University Press, 2010. Print.

Cossman, Brenda. *Sexual Citizens: The Legal and Cultural Regulation of Sex and Belonging*. Redwood: Stanford University Press, 2007. Print

Duggan, Lisa. *The Twilight of Equality? Neoliberalism, Cultural*

Politics, and the Attack on Democracy. Boston: Beacon Press, 2003. Print.

Epstein, Rachel ed. *Who's Your Daddy? And Other Writings on Queer Parenting.* Toronto: Sumach Press, 2009. Print.

Goldberg, Susan, and Chloë Brushwood Rose eds. *And Baby Makes More: Known Donors, Queer Parents, and Our Unexpected Families.* London: Insomniac Press, 2009. Print.

Golob, Alissa. "Why Are There Always Rainbow Flags at Pro-Abortion Rallies?" *Life Site News*, 16 September 2011. Web. 21 November 21 2014.

Kelly, Fiona. *Transforming Law's Family: The Legal Recognition of Planned Lesbian Motherhood.* Vancouver: University of British Columbia Press, 2011. Print.

Puar, Jasbir. *Terrorist Assemblages: Homonationalism in Queer Times.* Durham: Duke University Press, 2007. Print.

Serano, Julia. *Whipping Girl: A Transsexual Woman on Sexism and the Scapegoating of Femininity.* Emeryville: Seal Press, 2007. Print.

Smith, Miriam. *Political Institutions and Lesbian and Gay Rights in the United States and Canada.* New York: Routledge, 2008. Print.

Sullivan, Nikki. *A Critical Introduction to Queer Theory.* New York: New York University Press, 2003. Print.

11.
"Side by Side, Always and Forever"

CATHY DESCHENES

WHEN I WAS TWENTY-THREE and a half weeks pregnant with twins, I was at home with my two sons and felt my waters break. I was rushed by the ambulance to the hospital, where the doctors spent the next three days trying to stop labour each time it started. An ultrasound revealed our babies, Jordan and Katie, weren't doing well. They looked very weak, and their hearts weren't healthy. We were advised that once labour started, our babies wouldn't survive because of their prematurity and because they were very sick. We came to terms with this news and decided that we wanted to have a peaceful delivery and keep our babies with us. We asked that no resuscitative measurements be performed, since we knew the outcome would ultimately be the same. We set a plan in place and were ready to spend as much time as possible with our babies in our arms.

"HOW VERY SOFTLY YOU BOTH TIPTOED INTO OUR LIVES"

On November 16, after being awake off and on all night, I felt very ill. I had never felt this way before, as if I only felt the skin on my body and nothing else. My doctor arrived to see me, and once I described my symptoms, he knew it was time. As I had a fever and contractions, he advised me that an infection had started. Since my waters had been broken for three days, he knew that we would be delivering both babies that day. Just twenty four weeks pregnant and the day we had dreaded yet certainly longed for had arrived.

Since my previous labours were only a few hours, we thought this labour would also be quick. By 12:00 p.m., the contractions were picking up; I tried to focus and remember that no matter what the day's outcome was, this was their day, this was my day, and this was my birth.

I was surrounded with family members, friends, and my loving husband for the duration of my labour. I wanted to ensure I still had a natural childbirth, not only for my soon-to-be-born babies but also for me. It was very important to me that I was alert and attentive during the birth. I wanted to feel and remember every moment and, while this may sound strange to some, I personally didn't want to take any medication that might take away any of the experience.

As the afternoon progressed, the contractions became stronger. The nurses kept coming in and out of my room, offering me medication. I was so frustrated by this; they said that I should not feel pain because I was going to have a traumatic birth. I advised them that whether my babies lived or passed, I wanted a natural childbirth. I wanted to feel the pain. I wanted the full experience. Once I was firm and explained our wishes, I was fully respected and understood.

I continued to labour, and by 2:30 p.m., the contractions were more regular. I laboured in the Jacuzzi, in the bed, and on the birthing ball. By 3:20 p.m., things started picking up, and I knew the time was getting closer. The contractions were strong, almost unbearable. I advised the nurse to call the doctor, and then I sat on the bed rocking back and forth. I could feel Jordan sitting right there, but it was not time, as the nurse and doctor were not there.

I could not deliver yet, so I rocked back and forth thinking that as soon as the doctor arrived it would be time. I was not about to give in to the overwhelming pressure to push. I had to wait, and I knew they would be here soon. At 3:40 p.m., the doctor, a close family friend who saw us through this pregnancy, walked in. The timing was amazing. I did not want to have any other doctor deliver my precious babies.

Just then, in walked our favourite nurse, Kathleen. She had just come on shift, and all I could think about was there was someone watching over us; in that moment, to have the two professionals we needed the most be present meant so much. We had an amazing doctor and nurse in the room, and now our babies were about to arrive.

IT'S TIME TO MEET OUR BABIES

Dr. P., our obstetrician, sat on the edge of the bed. I told him it was time and he told me it would be all right. I felt at peace, even though I knew that our lives were about to change forever. I lay down very slowly, as the contractions were so intense. He prepared me for the birth and described exactly what was about to take place. Kathleen got a warm blue receiving blanket, and she placed it on my chest.

At 3:50 p.m., our son Jordan was born. He was placed on my chest. I cried. I was so excited to finally meet him, and then I realized that I would soon have to say goodbye. Dr. P. broke my waters for Katie. She was coming and nothing was stopping her. As I lay there staring at Jordan, I looked over at our doctor and asked him, "What's going on?"

He had a half smile on his face when he told me that Katie's foot was born first. He was holding her foot in his hand and asked me if I wanted to feel her foot. Right away I said, "Yes!" I reached down and held her tiny foot in my hand. The experience was overwhelming and something that I will never forget. I then knew it was time to push again.

At 4:02 p.m., Katie was born, footling breech. She was immediately placed onto my chest, where a warm pink blanket was waiting for her. I held both my precious babies and continued to cry. I remember saying out loud that life was so unfair. Dr. P. and Kathleen agreed. When I looked over to ask Kathleen what time the birth had taken place, I found her crying too. She could not get the words out. She could not tell me the times.

As I held both of my babies on my chest, all I could think about was the short time we were going to have together. My babies both took a few gasps of air, and they gently moved their arms. It would be those small movements that would affect us for the rest of our lives.

"ONLY AN HOUR YOU STAYED, BUT WHAT AN IMPRINT BOTH YOUR FOOTSTEPS HAVE BOTH LEFT UPON OUR HEARTS."

One of the most amazing memories I have from our time with Katie and Jordan is spending so much time with them in the hospital after their birth. I remember our nurse advising us that there was no "rush" to say good-bye. My feelings were torn, celebrating their births and mourning their deaths at the same time. I was not prepared to let them go; I wanted to keep them with us forever. That was the plan: to keep them forever. Yet we had to relinquish them at some point.

They told us to take our time. How much time I thought? "Take your time," was the BEST piece of advice the nurse could have offered us. We spent fourteen hours with our babies in our hospital room and had the opportunity to rock them in the rocking chairs. Family and friends came to see us and our babies. Our babies, too, had the opportunity to spend the night in our room with us. When we were "ready," saying goodbye was much easier.

MEMORIES

When we prepared to leave the hospital, the only things in my arms were two small memory boxes. These boxes contained very precious memories of our babies' short lives: handprints, bracelets, the measuring tape used to measure them both, their bonnets, etc.

Before going home, there were arrangements to be made. We arrived at the funeral home where we met with the funeral director. We gave him the obituary that I had written, and we then made all the arrangements for the visitation and the service. We made it known that we wanted our babies buried together. There was no other option for us; we would not separate them. They were to be placed side by side, as they had been for the past twenty-four weeks. Jordan was on my left side, Katie on my right. The funeral director looked at us and said, "I have the perfect little white coffin for them to share." We were at peace. The visitation and service were beautiful. All of Jordan and Katie's mementos from the hospital were shared with everyone. We were overwhelmed with the love and support that our friends and family had for us and our babies, Jordan and Katie. While we weren't able to introduce everyone to Jordan and Katie in the short time they were here with us, the visitation allowed us to share with them the memories that we did have.

SPECIAL OCCASIONS

Six months after their passing, we had an unveiling ceremony at the cemetery. This was a beautiful celebration where friends and family gathered and we unveiled their monument. We released balloons and homing doves and shared some stories about our babies' short life. Following this, we gathered together for an afternoon BBQ. It was a very nice way to celebrate their life.

Every year on Katie and Jordan's birthday, we take the day off work and school, and we have a "family day." Typically, the day consists of a visit to the cemetery, followed by a nice family dinner that our kids plan, with a special cake included. Over the years, several trips to the cemetery have involved releasing balloons with messages into the sky. One year, Joshua's special message was found a few days later in New York State by another grieving family.

"CARRYING YOU ON MY SHOULDERS"

Over the years, I learned to carry Jordan and Katie on my shoulders. This wasn't easy in the beginning and something I had to practice. I learned to accept the chirping of birds, the two doves that appeared around the house, the random things that happened in the house, and the times I saw twins in strollers, as signs that my precious babies were still here and with me.

Learning to cope with grief has been one of the toughest things I have ever had to experience. I went through a roller coaster ride of emotions: sadness, anger, rage, etc. I found that it's really important to accept each and every one of these feelings and embrace them, not hide them. It's important to cry and let it out, to talk to friends and family, or to seek professional advice or to find local support groups when the time is right, and not when someone says you should. People grieve at their own pace and in their own time. Everyone grieves at their own pace and in their own time.

Jordan and Katie are, and will always be, a part of me and my family.

"Until we meet again"—Mom.

12.
Tales of Survival from a Mother on the Edge

Listening to Love, Play and Creativity

CELESTE SNOWBER

I may have birthed you
but you have birthed me

ICOME TO THIS WRITING as a mother looking reflectively on the last twenty-four years of raising my twin sons and an older sibling in the midst of being a professor, scholar, poet, dancer, and single parent. My mothering has been inseparable from my other passions in life, and, at times, I felt I was barely surviving on the edge—I now see I thrived—and the edge became the centre. My passions, vocation, and mothering danced together and informed one another as I continually gave birth to what it means to be human in the soil of humour, creativity, and love.

I've never been very good at surfing, but there are perpetual waves one must ride in the raising of twins. One must enter the flow and ride the seas of motherhood and forego the best practices in parenting books. Those guidelines and instructions work when one is not tired: parenting multiples and being well rested are not usually partners. I often wonder how I survived raising identical twins without access to the kind of ergonomic strollers one has today that look more like racing bikes from Volvo than the contraptions in the early nineties. I found it so difficult getting both of my boys in that double big stroller and walking up the hill to bring their older brother to school, I just threw one in a backpack and the other in a snugly, and that was my workout. (Who really needed to go to the gym?) In fact, going to the gym would always raise my blood pressure: getting both children in and out of the car at the appropriate time and into an aerobics class. And once I entered, the ambience was akin to the fitness gurus commanding you to whip your body in shape, as if Captain Picard of the Starship Command were in charge of your body. My experience at the local gym was not a paradigm of listening to and honouring the body, which was deeply connected to my life as a dancer, as a scholar studying embodiment, and as a mother of three children—two being twins. The only thing I could do was to surrender to surfing the waves of my own life, which broke open a radical living in the present moment that no decades of a monastery or cloister could do. I often felt motherhood was a kind of monasticism; who needed to be woken up to chant or pray? I was woken up continually and invited into the practice of loving through everything. The holy in the ordinary was the order of my days and nights.

I rode those years out and went into full force. I spent countless hours attempting to tire my boys by playing on jungle gyms at the park, swimming at pools and lakes, making tent forts in our living room, wrestling on the floor, banging on pots and pans, and painting with our feet in the kitchen. We used both our handprints and footprints, which became far more interesting than regular footnotes. I dove into the physicality of being immersed in a sensory world through the eyes of my twins—Micah and Caleb, who often lived in a world of their own—and their singleton brother Lucas, four years older. I was an only child and have to admit that sometimes through my twins I was reminded of my dear parents, Frank and Grace, both arguing and loving with fiery passion. If I had believed in reincarnation, I would have thought my mom and dad came back in my twins.

I listened to all my children's noises, and since I could not dull them, or would even want to, I joined in and provided as much creativity and openness for all of us to celebrate the world of "play." My sons were my true teachers, even though I was simultaneously doing a PhD in the Faculty of Education and teaching undergraduates part time, when the twins were from three to seven-years old. I was being schooled into the aesthetics of the everyday—doctorate of living through the senses. No doubt, onlookers or neighbours looked at me with loathing at times, as I did not silence my children nor did I have all my ducks lined up in a row in my house or in my yard for that matter. I had an unraked and unmowed lawn, and of course, now there is a fancy ecological name for this wild behaviour. Who had time for such things?

Rakeless woman

I am a rakeless woman
burgundy and yellow
is strewn over bubble
concrete driveway
unmowed grass
clover green
laced with flaming
blood leaves

I don't have the heart
to sweep away
nature's collage
random art
on suburban lawn

We were busy dancing and singing, reading books, making up stories about Bozee the Slug, or climbing all over the stairs, furniture and couches. My son Micah now says, "Yes, my mother just produces creative machines." Now decades later he is an opera singer, his twin brother Caleb is a heavy metal musician and tattoo artist, and their older brother Lucas is a yoga teacher, marketer, and garlic farmer. I listened. I responded. Yes, I was overwhelmed at times! They came to me, and I was the student. I was more concerned with listening to the timbre of their souls, where the place of saying *yes* to life was forming, and going with it. I often felt as if I was not enough. I did not bake or have anything matching in my house, including their clothes for that matter, and even my older son Lucas asked at one point, "Mommy, could you bake like the other mothers, instead of writing books?" What saved me was my invitation to full-hearted play by the duo and singleton, who could not stop living and playing with the kind of bold curiosity that sages live with. Everything was a matter of delight. Even all the eggs cracking on the floor was a space for wonder. I don't even know how the dog survived, but thankfully our black lab, Pax, was forgiving of everyone pulling on her tail.

I can never forget the activity in my womb years ago, which I affectionately called the "womb studio," when Micah and Caleb, then named baby A and baby B, rolled and moved to the extent that it felt as if the World Cup were going on within my belly. The attention to the womb studio changed my life and initiated a whole way of attending to an inner life, which informed the integration of my life as scholar, mother, and artist. It is not that different now when my twins gather—the banter, back and forth in a way only twins know. But I have had a long-held fascination with how twins listen to each other and have a conversation of their own. Listening alone is a practice in life and necessary for writing and creating. They seem to have a privileged entrance to listening to each other. My task has always been to listen to the humour and wisdom in all situations; otherwise, I would have crumbled, especially as my path became one of being a single mom. The African proverb "it takes a village to raise a child" was often in my heart. I kept waiting for the village to show up while I raised the kids, but *we were the village,* and I now see, in retrospect, we were all catapulted into the curriculum of wonder. This was the curriculum of seeing and hearing beauty in the smallest occurrences and of having the ability to learn from tiny acts of dailiness, whether that was creating music on pots and pans, or making up stories, songs, and dances, or noticing birds and lying down to watch their flight path. I was continually invited into places of curiosity and awe by raising all my sons. The twins echo this reality in a chorus. The following poem, "A Song of Wisteria," reveals the thread of wonder woven into the fabric of our lives.

A Song of Wisteria

wisteria begs to be smelled
on rooftops of the carport
scents leak into our blue van
rushing in morning routine

kids in tow with a harried mother

    "Stop fighting, get your seatbelts on,
    don't transform the toy into a weapon—
    calm down,"

I say in my agitated voice
drooping wisteria interrupts us
my three sons stop their banter
pastel colors catch us all off guard
no one can miss the halt of beauty
my seven-year-old twins Micah and Caleb
proclaim, "Rainbow Flowers!"
naming gives the scent of belonging
they make up a song about the rainbow flowers
we all begin to sing it as a daily ritual
accompanying the drive to elementary school
saved by the sanity of aesthetics
our invitation to being awake
initiated by my singing duo

lavender petals remain on the windshield
fragrance releases through the death of the flower
pink wisteria and tears baptize my olive flesh
grief pours down my skin as my marriage is ending
a season of longing and releasing
each petal wrapped in the morning light
we do not hold creation—we are creation
each spider and song a map of beauty
no clear pattern for the map of the heart

wisteria knows when to bloom
my sons know when to sing
rainbow flowers form the chorus
to call us into our day
welcomed by a song of wisteria
and they are still singing.

The singing never stops, and the living curriculum integrates with my own scholarship and teaching to see and experience curriculum as lived rather than as just content. I continue to explore the arts as a place of inquiry. When one thinks of curriculum, it is often thought of as what subject (i.e., math, art, or languages). But there is a whole other curriculum happening on the margins of life—on the playground and in the hallways or what happens in unexpected moments of our lives. The "lived curriculum" has long been theorized by curriculum theorists in the field of education as a place where learning happens in the unexpected places. Here one is caught by surprise: knowledge and wisdom have the capacity to unfold in every corner of life. My research has been under the umbrella of arts-based research, which opens the space for poetic, performative, narrative, or visual ways of articulating scholarship. I continue to connect the autobiographical and artistic, personal and universal, in ways of listening to one's own life as a research practice. Immersing myself in the gift of motherhood has formed, transformed, and informed all the writing and performance; this immersion has also been central to my research in arts-based ways of inquiry over the last few decades. Motherhood was the yoga studio to train to be deeply awake to the curriculum of life.

The impulses of creativity my children had were honed and trained over the years, and now we have a family of sophisticated musicians and practitioners. My task in those years was to find small spaces of nourishment for solitude and remain faithful to my walking and writing practice every day, weaving them into the craziness of days.

Attending was the true writing studio, as being and living are the notes and chords of writing. I wrote and danced the world that lived me, and art was created out of immersion in dailiness. There were dances about laundry and letting go in order to integrate dance and story as a place of inquiry; there was a dissertation about the erotics of the everyday followed by essays connecting embodied ways of being, which wove themselves into books. Now it seems like a miracle, since I really don't know how I found the clarity of mind to write when I often could not find my keys.

Finding and Minding

there is too much finding
one could spend a lifetime
finding things, places, people
I am still trying to find misplaced
socks, misplaced objects,
and not to mention place,
a sense of place in the
endeavour of finding the right
mate, jobs for grad students,
universities for children,
publishers for books and then
there is the constant search
for good organic vegetables
and finding all the kinds of men
that I really end up looking for
which aren't the ones that
are working with their hands
in the way that I might really like
but the ones who can fix my shelves
the water heater, the roof, the
ant invasion, and it does seem that
they are usually if not always men
who come to the door, as I have called
them, and of course they always want
money to fix this or that and all the time
it is my heart that needs to be fixed
and once I really have gotten my heart fixed
there is one other item that breaks down
and this morning it was the brakes which
have already been fixed so many times
and once again I am in the finding mode
how long can one spend finding until you
are bone weary of finding and realize it
is because you were losing something in the
first place, or never really had it or wanted it
and one wonders if you really were a good

Buddhist if you wouldn't have to find anything
because there would be no attaching
and of course there is that well-known Christian scripture,
which I can't seem to find at the moment which says,
the lost will be found, but they were not really talking
about objects were they, and perhaps I have spent
way more time finding myself than objects in my life
thus I now am making a recommitment to losing,
loosening and decluttering and throwing
away. Less is more and I want more with less
after all that was the cookbook I used for years
and now I just want to shed everything I can
so there will be less finding and more minding
mindfulness instead of findfulness
we are in a state of findfulness on this planet
constantly seeking to be found, to find, to discover,
to come upon, which is the root of find, and of course
I am all for coming, but wouldn't it just be luxurious
not to be in a finding mode, and just remove the
(f) from finding and it would be inding.
Inding would be better than ending, because there
would be no need for finding even after the ending
and it could just be the place of no finding.
With inding one could just settle into a state of
restfulness that if you didn't find the object,
plan, person, desire, fulfillment, vision, vegetable
or job it really wouldn't matter, because that
would be the goal in and of itself. But then would
have to find the inding and be mindful and the whole
cycle would just start again, eventually one would
be just left with a few letters, leaning into a
syllabic praise which defies anything to find or mind.

For years, I truly felt like a "mother on the edge," juxtaposed
with surprises of immense beauty, difficulty, joy, and laughter.
My parents were passed from this earth; I was thousands of miles
from family and had little support. I drew as much community
around as I could, but the sheer fatigue and hormonal fluctuations

through peri-menopause can be a recipe for fragility. I wrote out of that vulnerability every morning, early before my kids went off to school or after I dropped them off and before going to the university. Thousands of pages adorned my moleskin notebooks, and eventually ideas were formed for chapters, essays, poetry, and books connecting my research on embodiment and the arts. My journal was my lover, accepting all of me in any form and always being there to receive a fresh release of blood to ink. I now see the edge was the centre. I went to the precipice and was summoned to not only let go but to let be. Artmaking and living are inextricably connected, and one cannot exist without the other.

There is a lot of talk about the edge being the centre, but nothing puts you faster on the edge than a combination of lack of sleep and multiple tasks, where you feel your limitations are a bold colour in all of your life as raising multiples. Of course, the joy is multiplied, but all the reading material and theorizing cannot substitute for a theorizing through the flesh. I lived in the realm of multiples as there was more laundry, more tears, and more joy. I often thought of all the research about multiple intelligences, but nothing prepares for living a multiple life more than twins.

Precipice Wisdom

she is living on a precipice
fast raising brilliance
on the other side of rain
last edge of summer
she wants to jump off, glide over,
through, above, under, in
the arms that could hold
her with a kind of space
which breathes through the cedar
salt that finds room for water in ocean
she'll run her fingers through the green moss
on the tree which she has loved for years
twined trees from the trunk
sky bound from their birth
those trees know her

as one who lives
in multiples:
twins, loves, books, pets
orgasms and spasms
tears and laments
deaths and births
keep coming in multipli/cities
the land grounds her
in edges of flight
the only precipice to jump from
is to once again walk the path
in relentless gentleness
and find tender

There was a school of learning to live poetically, artistically, and improvisationally in the class of mothering. The multiplicity of life beckoned a thinking on the feet, yet even though I was mothering multiples, I saw them as individuals. One of the most important things I could do as a parent was to see the glimmers of how each of my children's souls would emerge, and it was my role to cheer them on, where I saw these flickers. Flickers come where we experience joy as humans. Listening to joy can be a huge detector in what we are called to do on this planet, whether it is the thrill of organizing LEGO bricks, making up songs, relating to others, or climbing trees. Childhood had a kind of studio feel in my house, and exploration was a food group; we partook every day in the glory of textures, sounds, movements, and colours. Creativity was central to ways of living and being. Therefore, to dress my twins in uniform ways, or cultivate sameness, went against everything I believed in and treasured. I watched for how they would evolve and encouraged them to be their own individual beings, filled with the differences of sensibilities and senses. Each created his own sentences into this world.

Twins are a phenomenon. Every parent of multiples knows how people stare, talk, and wonder about what this is truly like. It is hard to imagine that years ago twins would be dressed the same and not encouraged to inhabit their unique selves. My twins made an extra special effort to be different. If one got an earring in the ear, the other got one in the opposite ear, and then both ears. I will never forget when Micah and Caleb wanted the hair stylist to shave M on the back of one head, and C on the back of the other head, as we were going to a big family reunion. They announced their uniqueness from the clothes they wore to the style of music they listened to. I made a decision a long time ago as a parent not to waste energy concerning decisions about hair, and I let them choose what was important to them, whether it was tattoos or piercings or the colours they loved. I had bigger problems to solve such as the roof falling apart, paying the bills, and resolving sibling rivalry. And there was certainly plenty of squabbles, but always there was wonder. We all wandered into wonder together.

Listening to Love

delight of multiplicities
where two voices become five
and math is an exercise in joy
a team of two can shake worlds
move furniture and hearts
with twenty fingers and four eyes

you my twins
have always been shining stars
individual and collective
working in a trio with your brother
who glowed with you in the earth and sky

you each lived in galaxies
a constellation of surprise
poured through our lives
in unfolding awe
I may have birthed you
but you have birthed me
opened the place for wonder
a love unequaled in this journey
multiples were not only twins
but multiples were all of you—

Micah, Caleb, and Lucas
a force unto your own

December called you to be born
three days from one another
and I still bare the miracle
of being your mom
and you have been my mentor
in listening to love

People often ask me, "How did you do it?" How did I raise twins and another older son, while going through tenure, having a demanding profession, writing, dancing, mothering, cooking, and attending lacrosse, hockey, baseball, soccer games, theatre and music performances, and being the home that all the teenagers gravitated to? I am not sure how I did it myself, but the only real truth that sustains is that of a fierce love. Fierce love accompanies children as soon as they are in the womb and come out to the world. These tales are tales of love, and they reveal more than survival. I did not only survive, I thrived. Perhaps a new term needs to be born called *surthrival*! Multiple births and multiple loves. Here is a tale to be told.

13.
Naming the Planets

JESSICA JENNRICH

I SIT AT OUR KITCHEN table helping my son name the planets. A homework assignment he pulled from the bottom of his book bag and placed on the table between us. It is crumpled and covered with the debris of young boys: crumbs and pencil smears, chewing gum and eraser dust.

It is April, and spring has been coaxed out of the ground reluctantly. Errant piles of snow defiantly remain under the shade of tall pine trees and in dark corners. I shake out the wrinkled paper and begin the task of helping my seven-year-old son name the planets. He balances on the edge of a chair, impossibly skinny and already resistant. Homework is its own form of torture to him. He prefers to dig his small capable hands deep into the earth and catalog the insects that slither forth. Or to traverse the mangroves at the edge of our river to catch an elusive glimpse of the mysterious water snake who often bursts forth at sunset. He knows more about reptiles and zoology than I ever will but struggles to form letters that face the right direction.

I point to the paper as the planets line up in a neat row sized in relation to the butter-yellow sun and named after Roman gods whose stories I never heard. His brother and sister, twins born almost five years ago to the day, bat oblong birthday balloons—prepared for their party to be held later today—past his head while we try to work. I explain that the planets don't line up so cleanly above our heads, looking less and less like the pristine march of circles his fingers impatiently drum over. I tell him the planets twirl like a double helix roiling through the cosmos at dizzying speeds and unimaginable distances from Earth while his fingers jump from planet to planet on the page and use them like some kind of intergalactic stepping-stones. I point to the sky as I talk, trying to generate excitement and mystery, and implore him to stop tapping his pencil on the table and imagine the vast cosmos above us. As a balloon sails past his head, he sighs and tells me that in space there is no sound; this, I suppose, is knowledge.

We give up and surrender to the sunshine and the birthday preparations. I'm tired of pretending to care about the sky beyond what we can see. I am slipping into my annual state of depression that arrives with a bang on each and every birthday of these twins, like a tax collector pounding down my door for debts. I don sunglasses and begin arranging cake and filling helium balloons, hoping I can distract the twins from the sharp fact that no one but us is coming to this party. Briefly, their other mother and I had considered throwing a huge party with personalized invitations at some elaborate child-themed location but thought better. It is with a resigned loneliness we chose a party with just the five of us instead of facing the inevitable rejection of an entire classroom of children or perhaps even worse—a party filled with forced attendees, uncomfortable smiles, and a mechanical rendition of *Happy Birthday* as a finale. No, we thought, better to save our heartbreaks for something worthwhile.

When the party suffers its last gasp and the five of us have wrung all the cheer possible out of this affair, I think again of the planets and decide to name my own. My own planets are hard to pin to paper, impossible to measure and plot, avoid and attract, insistent on bowling through our lives with frequency and proximity beyond my control. The warm spring breeze that flutters the leaves over the mud puddles in our driveway inspires magic. If the ground can produce flowers whose petals poke through the ice crust still present on the dark side of the garden, then couldn't my planets be just as real as those untouchable orbs of ice and rock spinning around the sun in endless circles?

I name the first planet Joy. Joy's surface gleams like a marble as she rolls across the icy ground to help me sculpt a dragon out of the last remaining snow. She ran in circles around my head five years ago when I laughed helplessly at the ultrasound image of not one, but two babies dancing in my belly. She flutters past and pulls my hands from flipping a page in a book to holding tiny hands instead. She rolls smoothly across the boring beige carpet and transforms me into a growling and snarling monster that chases my children, screaming with laughter, when I capture them and tickle them until they wiggle away. Joy blows bubbles that show me a future as seamless and shiny as blown glass and reminds me of lazy summer days spent with two newborns and a toddler, rocking their warm bodies cradled tightly over my heart. Joy flashes by in Christmas bulbs and in the glass of an aquarium filled with glowing jellyfish. In her refection, I can see every first smile.

I name the next planet Fear whose fur sticks to my sweater no matter the effort I make to remove it. She tangled herself into my hair one April five years ago on the birthday of these twins when Joy rolled out the door. She plunged into my mouth and wound round my tongue making me unable to speak when I thought something may be wrong with our newborn daughter. Fear looped around my feet making the seven steps it took from our daughter's hospital bed to the MRI imaging room endless, playing on repeat for eternity. Fear coiled around my wrists and pulled my face toward the screen and pried my eyes wide so that nothing could erase the black blotches the doctor showed me on our daughter's nine-month-old brain, "an old stroke from birth," the doctor said as Fear's locks of hair knotted into a ball incapable of ever being untangled. Her tendrils are endless and spin into a tight sphere whose landscape can grow no vegetation, can host nothing but fiberes that mat themselves into tight itchy plains always ready to be deployed.

Frustration is the planet who throws herself under my tires, tossing me into drifts of pristine glittering snow. Frustration screams around corners as our daughter bashes her hand, the one that refuses to uncurl, into the bars of the swing set, shouting how she hates her hand, hates this stroke, hates everything. Frustration's siren deafens every possible note of a song, making it so I can merely whisper tunelessly our daughter's walking song that an eager physical therapist suggested I sing when she was barely two. I gathered our daughter up from the ground for the hundredth time and began marching her chubby legs, clad in bulky plastic leg braces and tied to an elaborate harness, round and round our home, frustration shrieking past us, drowning out my cheery tune. Frustration is the sand in my shoes and the almost that never was. Frustration is days spent on hold with insurance companies, doctors' offices, and therapists who speak in vague language about a someday that may never be. The ground of Frustration is littered with discarded leg braces and beads of sweat dropped from our daughter's brow as she works. Works to open her hand, take a step, sit up, hold her lunch tray, zip her coat, brush her hair, explain over and over to her preschool classmates why she moves differently, why her hand will not open, why she wears that leg brace. Frustration moves so fast she ignites a trail of smoke behind her, whipping past our home, singeing the tips of our fingers and then screaming by with only the smell of smoke in our noses and the desire to lock our doors. We wait to hear her howling in the distance, bracing ourselves, but are helpless nonetheless for when she decides to arrive.

The planet Pain slices through the skin of our daughter's tendons as the doctors work to "fix" her, to make her look "normal." Pain is dirty and dry, pointy and sharp. She grows nothing but long ropes of briar bushes that embed under your skin. Pain rattles and bounces like a dancing skeleton and laughs a brittle cackle. Pain clatters and clunks into our home picking and pulling at our daughter's limbs, making her entire left side either too tight or too loose. Pain pretends to be a friend, rasping "if you make her stand like this" or "if you just spent more time stretching" and knows all along she has nothing to offer but lies. Pain beams light into my iris and sends shock waves thudding inside my head in hospital waiting rooms in three states in just five years. Pain knew no matter how many new adventures our battered little family tried that there would be no escape. She tells me "children's brains are like plastic" and promises I can make my daughter better when she knows it is all pointless. Pain likes the taste of the tears I leak onto her barren planet floor when I fail over and over again to answer my daughter as she asks me "Why?"

I name the planet who froze my daughter's body and gathered an electrical storm in her brain on the day of her birth Cruelty. Her surface is a sponge of clouds battered by lightening. It is impossible to land anywhere on Cruelty without a voltage so strong it will shock you insane. Cruelty collects her clouds and revs her engines into waiting ears. She pretends to light my way towards a new job or a new friend only to overload her own circuits and destroy it all just for a lark. Cruelty changes her shape and hides, always waiting for me to forget about her so she can surprise me with a storm of destruction. Her vivid flashing, not unlike a neon bar sign, makes our friends' eyes blind to our family. The storm she conjures leaves us illuminated for onlookers to watch as they pass by—"what a shame," they say, "she could have been so pretty"—as we rummage make-shift shelters to survive her blows. We speak of the damage Cruelty has wreaked only in whispers after too much wine, when we look at the artifacts of our former lives and wonder whether we will survive her next strike.

The planet Sorrow knocks on my window, clicking the glass with a gnarled hand that looks just like my daughter's. Sorrow stops time as I turn over and over the ballet shoes our daughter wants but cannot have while she stands in the middle of a bustling department store, appearing to others a woman possessed. Sorrow has thick branches populated with wet leaves that free themselves to plaster the side of our car as we drive from doctor to doctor, from city to city. At the bus stop, our daughter stands alone and tries to talk to the other little girls who turn away silently and gaze instead at the leaves blowing past. Sorrow knows she has won when our daughter stops trying to make friends anymore, when she takes up talking to her dolls about growing up and being like everyone else instead. Sorrow is forever a frozen dark night that sends a chill into my core, impossible to shake no matter how many blankets I burrow under. Sorrow grows her territory, expanding her geography to slip into the blank spaces between the words I type to pretend everything is just fine. Soon my ghosts will show up in keystrokes instead of footsteps. Sorrow is haunted by a thousand wrong turns and mistakes that come to visit me night after night of thin sleep. She is circled by a moon named Regret and the two of them revolve around each other in a sinister dance that covers my world in a haze of shadows that creep into the food I eat, the words I say, the air I breathe. Sorrow likes me on my knees.

Laugher is a planet who hides under my tongue and shows up at the most inopportune times. In a meeting, I remember something far away and hide my chuckle with a cough. Laughter is a pure planet, glowing bright blue, and never far from my reach. She is indiscriminate in her humour and causes me to guffaw, as the twins model lingerie fetched from my drawer, and to snort at the hypocrisy of a country that makes our love illegal but sells guns at the grocery store. Laughter wants to be touched; her surface is buoyant like a ball and begs to be bounced. A cocked eyebrow from my partner during a parent teacher conference makes her appear, and I giggle like a preteen girl, still flirting after fifteen years. Laugher fits into my pocket and there she stays, ready to bounce out and drip happy tears from my tired eyes, just when I think I couldn't ever smile again.

Love is the last planet I name. Love zooms through the air showering the ceiling with sparks that fall onto our shoulders. Love is a planet of particles. Love's glitter affixes itself to my skin and her sparkling detritus scatters itself over everything. It isn't unusual to find piles of Love hidden under our daughter's bed when I kiss her good night and fold her limbs under her covers. Love is a pinprick of light when all that can be seen is unrelenting dark. Love brightens our eyes and her twinkle is so brilliant she can outshine any planet in this fairytale solar system should the wind happen to blow just right.

I wheel the trash, overflowing with wrapping paper and extinguished candles, to the curb later that same night and hurry with my task. Finally, having finished helping my son with his forgotten homework, it is now late and the spring weather has retreated back towards winter. Someone once said April was the cruelest month, and I think he was certainly right. I stop, as the cold curls around my feet, and stare above at the night sky. The real planets are out there I am sure, but mine are too, so I stop and name my planets.

14.
Milkshake Lovers, Unite!

Performing Infant Feeding:
A Narrative of Theory and Practice

TERRI HAWKES

IWOULD LIKE TO SHARE a good ol' family recipe that I have been testing:

Infant Feeding Milkshake

Mix one part theory and one part practice in baby bottle, add a delicate dash of breast milk (fresh or pumped), a smidge of formula, a cup full of feminist theories, a healthy dose of mother and non-mother love, and vigorously shake all ingredients to yield a tasty infant feeding "milkshake."

In so mixing, I join the recipe sharing of theorists who honour the value of personal experience, especially how such experience might be contextualized next to thoughtful theoretical analysis of the cultural and ideological underpinnings of "infant feeding." I view "infant feeding" as a variable recipe that could include any or all ingredients such as breast milk, formula, alternative milks and/or pureed solids, which can be dispensed by many combinations of caregivers. Alison Bartlett, among others, advocates theorizing from experience, and suggests that "breastfeeding is as much a product of current cultural perceptions as it is a personal 'decision'" (3). In this paper, I will draw on my previous academic research "The Millennial Wean (Performing Breastfeeding in the Global North: 1989–2013)" as well as my personal experience of feeding twin infants, which consisted almost entirely of breastfeeding. My goal is not to weigh in on particular sides of the infant feeding debates but to share my findings while advocating for informed access to choice. To that end, I will contextualize my autoethnographic experiences of infant feeding alongside current theoretical discourse on the subject. The results should yield a frothy full-bodied milkshake for the reader's leisurely consumption.

INGREDIENT LIST

a) Theory

As a basis for my theoretical analysis of current ideologies and practices of infant feeding, I refer to twelve scholarly texts on this subject all written between 1989 and 2013, a period I refer to as the "Millennial Wean." I suggest that the Millennial Wean is now a moment in twenty-first-century maternal studies when academics recognize the delicious developments achieved in maternal infant feeding theories and practices in the twentieth century while they simultaneously wean themselves from the comforting thought that the mission is over. Concurrently, as one of those feminist academics, I would like to actively acknowledge the growth still needed in the areas of *awareness, education, and access*. I would like to add my singular voice to the academic and mainstream publications asking academics, medical practitioners, social workers, and mothers to increase their *awareness* of various perspectives and options around infant feeding. I am appreciative of the opportunity for this publication and for the multimedia platforms that are emerging to contribute to *education* around mothering and infant feeding, and I would hope that this discourse finds its way not only to academic institutions but also to social and health support systems for families. My wish is that the printed volume and electronic versions of this anthology might facilitate a discourse that contributes to increased *access* to a greater number of infant feeding choices for a wider spectrum of mothers.

One small contribution towards awareness could come through an examination of publications in this field. Thus, my first aim is to provide a textual analysis of what I have here identified as six major areas that resonate as central issues in twenty-first-century discourse around breastfeeding. These areas are breastfeeding in private versus public spheres; the medicalization of infant feeding;

the sexualization of breastfeeding; the social construction of the "good mother"; milk sharing and/or replacement feeding; and one of the earliest (and most inescapable) feminist issues—essentialism. Fodder for my analysis will include scholarly texts alongside mainstream-popular publications.

Collectively, the dozen academic texts I have synthesized here speak to a myriad of issues, including the following: feminist empowerment, poverty, medicalization of infant feeding, commoditization of infant food, public policy, replacement feeding, sexualization of breastfeeding, choice, sacredness, strategic essentialism, feminist theory, feminist practice, public breastfeeding, superiority of breastfeeding, social construction of breastfeeding, breast milk exchange, and the globalization of biomedical values. Dialogue around the essentialist constructions of mothers—or the notion that mothers are "born" to perform the social and practical role of "mother" in a prescribed way—is discussed in texts by La Leche League (LLL), Hausman (*Mother's Milk*), and Van Esterik. The works of Bartlett, Giles (*Fresh Milk*), Carter, and O'Reilly ("Introduction," *Mother Outlaws*) further reveal the complexity of this contentious topic and contribute to my aim of using strategic essentialism in order to emancipate women from a lack of choices related to mothering practice, in particular, infant feeding.

Bartlett, Giles ("Fountains"), Carter, and LLL highlight maternal sexuality, a realm I extend to include the importance of the sensuality of infant feeding. Carter and Blum lead the charge in challenging the medicalization of infant feeding, while Giles (*Fresh Milk*) and Bartlett join my quest for mothers to have more opportunities to make informed choices about the way(s) that they feed their children. Arguments that the "good mother" and "intensive mothering" constructions undermine mothers' agency reverberate in the texts of Thurer, Hays, and Maushart. The history of "milk sharing" and the commoditization of infant feeding are recorded by Carter, Blum, and Hausman (*Mother's Milk*), who also examine current public policies in this area. Giles delineates the importance of the inclusion of "herstories" (stories told by women—as opposed to "histories"—stories traditionally told by men) in efforts to share mothers' experiences of infant feeding (*Fresh Milk*); both Bartlett and Giles (*Fresh Milk*) validate my desire to frame my research using the lenses of personal experience and academic investigation simultaneously. Issues arising from the divide between public and private roles in terms of gendered forms of labour and the resulting limits on mothers' choices about infant feeding abound in virtually all of these scholarly texts, most notably in Smith, Hausman *(Mother's Milk)*, Labbok, Bartlett, and Blum. Many suggest much-needed solutions to combat this persisting and detrimental social construction, which supports my notion that blurring the public and private boundaries will aid women in expanding their infant feeding choices. While they originate from diverse experiences and focus on various different aspects of mothers and infant feeding, the texts that I have chosen align with and support my call for awareness, education, and access.

In a continued quest to contribute to increased awareness of the current dialogues around infant feeding, I shift from an analysis of scholarly literature towards a review of a number of "mainstream go-to" books, meant to illuminate conscientious mothers of the new millennium. These works include publications by Elizabeth Noble, Martha and William Sears, Benjamin Spock, Burton White, and Penelope Leach, all of which have been published or revised within the last two decades, with the exception of Mr. White's volume, written in 1985. Burton White offers a reasoned account of the evolution of infant feeding in North America between the early 1900s and 1985, and he concludes that there is enough medical evidence to "recommend to all new parents that they attempt prolonged breastfeeding if it is at all possible … [it is] clearly the preferred method" (266). Elizabeth Noble, often referred to by parents of multiples, states "Breast-feeding is the simplest, cheapest, and most convenient way to feed twins, triplets, and quadruplets … every attempt should be made to support the mother in the ways described here so that enough milk is produced even for super-twins … I strongly advise breast-feeding" (250-259). Her position places responsibility for infant feeding on the mother, and she urges mothers to adopt the practice of breastfeeding. Noble suggests that if supplemental feedings are required, there is an opportunity for paternal involvement. Penelope Leach offers logical points for the advantages of both breastfeeding and bottle-feeding, although she encourages mothers who start by breastfeeding to leave their options open. Ultimately, she weighs in on the side of choice: "If there is a decision to be made about whether a baby is to be breast-fed, it has to be the mother's because she is the only person in the world who can act on it: it is her body, her lifestyle and specifically her mothering rather than interchangeable parenting that is primarily in question" (Leach 55).

The seventh edition of Benjamin Spock's *Dr. Spock's Baby and Child Care* advocates for breastfeeding and suggests an "essential" link with nature, "new knowledge about the physical and emotional advantages, partly to the general respect among the young for nature and the desire to do things the natural way. We are beginning to see more babies from lower-income and minority families being breast-fed. I hope this trend will continue" (106). However, Spock's perspective does not explain how double income earning or single-parent families might make breastfeeding work if circumstances prove too challenging, "If you've got the determination to succeed and to gain the emotional support for your breast-feeding at work and at home, then working and breast-feeding can both succeed, no matter what your schedule or situation" (116). Long considered the gurus of attachment parenting and breastfeeding, Martha and William Sears make a very compelling case for breastfeeding, citing numerous physical and psychological advantages for both the mother and the child. Ultimately, though, they start with the same assumptions as their colleague, Dr. Grantly Dick-Read, who argues that "The newborn baby has only three demands. They are warmth in the arms of its mother, food from her breast, and security in the knowledge of her presence. Breastfeeding satisfies all three" (Reid qtd. in Sears 18). These are the basic premises that I absorbed from mainstream parenting literature, agreed with, and adopted during my breastfeeding years. I will now interrogate these positions alongside feminist infant feeding theories and my personal experience of the subject matter.

b) Practice

With that long list of academic and mainstream ingredients in mind, I offer my own personal favourite ingredients in the form of my experience of infant feeding during the Millennial Wean. My practice of infant feeding provoked personal reflections around the same themes as those that I have isolated in the scholarly texts, even though I could not have identified them as such at the time. Ultimately, I hope to synthesize the personal and theoretical by honouring personal experience as a mode of theorizing and archiving and by continuing to extend theories generated by other feminist academics in the area of infant feeding practices and ideologies. In addition to this, I share my mother's love of a good, thick milkshake!

EQUIPMENT LIST

The blender for this milkshake is informed by the personal positioning of me—the author. I am writing as an able-bodied, white, Anglo, heterosexual, academic, theatre practitioner and mother of fifteen-year old twins—from the decidedly privileged perch of white, middle-upper-class North Toronto. However, my position of relative privilege does not negate the legitimacy of my experiences. I believe that they are deserving of attention (as are all other perspectives), since the issue of infant feeding affects all of us at some point(s) in our lives, whether as a child or adult who will become a parent. This chapter represents a single voice from the middle-class Global North, although it is my hope that it will reverberate in other spheres and form a lactose link to my global sisters, as they experience a wide variety of milkshake recipes.

DIRECTIONS: CHOOSE FROM INGREDIENTS TO VARY FLAVOUR

Flavour One: "Essential" Eggnog

Most scholars reviewed here believe that there is a basis to essentialism as connected to breastfeeding, when essentialism is viewed as the "natural" ability of a woman to produce breast milk. Where the theorists start to differ is in the debate over whether or not infant feeding is a task that only women can carry out. Breaking this down into components of work, body, and performance, let us examine the possibilities. Most commonly, women do the physical production of breast milk[1]; however, the female need not be the mother of the child and the breast milk can be pumped by a mother and fed to infants by a parent or other caregiver. Thus, with regard

227

to work, I propose that with the proper support systems in place, the practice of feeding breast milk to infants can be shared work and is not always biologically determined. With regard to the body, the most common feminist position is that women should be able to make their own choices around the use of their body. Although some mainstream writers argue that there really is no choice other than to breastfeed (La Leche League; Sears) I concur with a number of other authors who have shown that it is a complex "choice" mediated by social, cultural, political, geographical, religious, economic, medical, emotional, familial, and practical circumstances (Bartlett; Carter; O'Reilly, "Introduction," *Mother Outlaws*). Thus, I conclude that the "choice" and ability to provide breast milk is not solely a question of biological determinism; a number of circumstances may affect infant feeding practices and may involve caregivers of any gender.

Around the issue of performance, I refer to Judith Butler's position that gender is performative. Butler argues that one should not assume that gender is an essential biological way of acting, but rather that "an internal essence of gender is manufactured through a sustained set of acts, posited through the gendered stylization of the body ... [thus] ... one that we anticipate and produce through certain bodily acts" (Butler xv-xvi). Thus, I suggest, by extension, a woman becomes "mother" through her repetitive actions, actions that could include breastfeeding, bottle feeding, diaper changing, hugging, comforting, educating, dressing, bathing, encouraging, protecting, etc.[2] Scholars that support this theory of gender performativity, who suggest that mothering is partially a social construction, might identify themselves as "non-essentialist" (Bartlett and Shaw; O'Reilly, "Introduction", *Twenty-first-Century*). At the other end of the spectrum, women are positioned as the only ones who can perform the role of mother (LLL; Hausman, (*Mother's Milk)*; Van Esterik). An alternative position balances biomedical and social-political influences—often called "strategic essentialism" (Blum; Carter; Giles, *Fresh Milk*). In this case, women could choose to use the argument of essentialism in a strategic manner when useful to support their choices around infant feeding.

My personal experience of over a decade ago positioned me as an "accidental essentialist," although I could not have identified

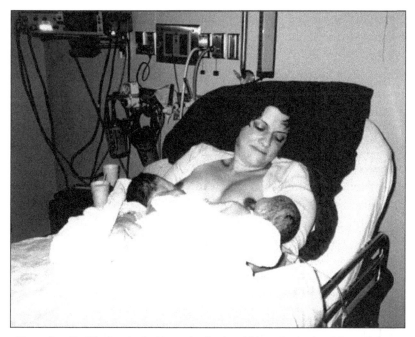

Figure One. Terri Hawkes (author) breastfeeding her children shortly after delivery. Toronto. 2000. Joanne Hawkes, photographer.

it as such at the time. I was a new-millennium mother of twins who planned to return to the workforce as soon as possible after giving birth. In retrospect, reflecting on the medicalized and arms-full image of me in the photo above, I should have projected that returning to paid employment might take longer than I imagined. The successful career that I had built for two decades (acting, writing, and directing) had its own set of rules. I was concerned about shift-work schedules and business travel, although I was determined to "have it all." When I was seven-months pregnant with twins a variety of challenges led me to temporarily curtail directing, writing, and on-camera acting, but I was still actively working as a voiceover actor for animation, radio drama, and commercials. Although not as intense as the other forms of work I often engaged in, it was still a challenge to do voice work—my full term nausea was an ordeal, breathing was demanding, sound engineers had to be creative with my newfound distance from the microphone, and my girth necessitated my use of the freight eleva-tor in one building. However, with the support of my colleagues,

I proudly soldiered on and provided my employers with what I trusted was seasoned and high-quality work.

One of my contract employers—a producer, with whom I had worked for over a year as an advertising spokesperson for a major retail chain—severed my contract immediately after I gave birth, possibly scared that I would be unable to fulfill my obligations. I would have loved to continue with this familiar and lucrative voice job, contributing to the financial care of my new children. Social assumptions of my "essential" indispensability to my children perhaps limited my opportunities here. I did complete a few animation voice jobs within weeks of giving birth to twins, thanks to flexible producers, voice directors, and a caregiver who travelled to sound studios with me so that I might nurse every one and a half to two hours. Nevertheless (with a partner who was often absent due to a demanding travel schedule), the role of parenting two babies was more challenging than I had anticipated.

I recall one particularly memorable film job that I received when my kids were four years old. They were both home sick with our third paid caregiver of the day, while my partner was out of town and I was committed to an overnight film shoot. It was the last on-camera job that I would accept. Concerned for the well-being of my children, I voluntarily gave up many job opportunities for non-paying yet flexible non-profit work and community and education boards. From my privileged position as the partner of a financially secure film executive, I reasoned that in taking on volunteer work I could determine my working hours and make what I perceived to be a valuable contribution to our community and our children's development. What I did not thoroughly process was how I was starting to contribute to my own diminishing career possibilities by taking nearly a decade's absence from the paid workforce. To clarify—I did not nurse my children for ten years. Not even two years. I breastfed my children until the age of fifteen months, at which point I was advised by doctors to give up the practice for my own health; they deemed that my prolonged breastfeeding of two children was contributing to my bone density loss. Even that was a hard "letting go" for me.

What I now realize was that the intense togetherness and bonding that came from fifteen months of full-time nursing and care of two children led me to be the "expert" on childrearing in our family. Prior to that, my partner and I had been equally inept. We learned together, fashioning a late-night routine of shared breastfeeding; every couple of hours throughout the night, we would stagger down the hall with two babes in arms to the couch in my office, which doubled as a breastfeeding station. My partner, Jeff, would pass each child to me, as I helped the babies latch on, "football hold" style. Jeff would return to bed, and an hour later, I would use the walkie-talkie to wake him. He would fumble down the hall again and take and change each baby one at a time, while I returned to bed. A couple of hours later, we started the routine again. Jeff was indispensable as a partner and father during those early weeks of all-night feedings. But he soon resumed his business travel, often leaving me to be the sole full-time parent.

Through exposure, experience, and the work of mothering, I became quite a capable parent. When Jeff was not travelling, he often worked evenings, and I was the de facto "parent in charge." All this to say that my personal experience was that breastfeeding for a prolonged length of time equipped me with skills that both my partner and I would then unconsciously use to determine that I was the more capable parent. As a result, we both felt I should have the responsibility of being the primary caregiver to our children, even after we had finished the breastfeeding stage. Although Jeff was a true partner in spirit for those early years, he was still out of town many days a month, so I gratefully received occasional help when we had visits from out-of-towners like Jeff's parents, my parents, and my grandmother. Our children's co-caregiver, Eva, continued to be in and out of our lives on a part-time basis for a number of years while she managed responsibilities to her own growing family. However, during that first year of parenting, Eva was truly a co-parent with me five days a week, feeding me while I produced and shared milk for two and helping me to manage the care of two infants for many hours a day.

Thus, I would assess that my (somewhat) unconscious embracing of full-time mothering was shaped by a number of forces: my skittish employer, my career-focused partner, my modelling of intensive mothering, and by the absence of my family in the Toronto area. These forces bolstered my emotional position that no one could do the job of parenting our children better than I could, leading me to a position of accidental essentialist. At the time, I was not aware enough to adopt a position that might have helped me retain a stronger foothold in my chosen profession. In hindsight, and with a few years of critical thinking under my belt, I now consciously support the notion of strategic essentialism while still acknowledging my gratitude for the opportunities that I had to be with my children. Today, I argue that other than the actual production of breast milk, the work of parenting can be learned and shared, and any capable parent or caregiver can facilitate the work of infant feeding. I argue for a model of "educated strategic essentialism," which honours a mother's self-knowledge and right to contribute to choices that she deems are best for her family.

Flavour Two: Sexual and Sensual Spice

In the contemporary Global North, the sexualization of non-maternal female breasts and the propensity to view mothers and pregnant women as non-sexual beings interfere with an acceptance of public breastfeeding, affecting the choices of mothers in both the private and public spheres. The scholars examined here concur in recognizing a traditional binary between the sexualized (non-maternal) breast and the non-sexual (lactating) breast. Although La Leche League makes efforts to assuage the fears of women by confirming that sexual feelings during lactation are normal in the privacy of one's home, the other academic texts examined here seem to unilaterally call for a re-examination around social norms of sexuality. The sexuality of the lactating breast that they refer to is not only mother to child but also adult to adult (Giles, "Fountains"). Some theorize about maternal sexuality beyond the heterosexual normative model (Giles, "Fountains"; Bartlett). Most suggest that power exists in embracing the sexuality of the maternal and that agency and sexuality can be discovered in autonomy and choice. Some scholars propose that higher self-esteem can be earned through sexualized actions that mothers choose to engage in and enjoy, including breastfeeding. Carter, Blum, Giles ("Fountains," *Fresh Milk*), and Bartlett argue against the social regulations around sexuality, and Bartlett calls for the value of mothers to be increased in our social economy.

My personal journey along the maternal sexual spectrum goes back to my first and only unplanned pregnancy. I was with my current partner at that time and was engaged in a healthy sexual relationship when my intrauterine device failed. The lovemaking at Lake Louise was sexy, the feeling of fertility was sexy, but the miscarriage that followed was not sexy. In fact, there was nothing sexy about the next six planned pregnancies and miscarriages. The frequent trips to the miscarriage specialists and clinics, the daily hormonal injections, the self-injected subcutaneous blood thinning needles, the trips to emergency, and the dilation and curettage (d & c) procedures were not sexy. Even an attempted insemination process was not sexy. It involved a small medical office for my partner equipped with pornographic magazines, a hospital bed with stirrups for me—you get the picture. So imagine my surprise when—after three years of medical appointments, and well into three months of bed rest, injections, and ultrasounds—I was successfully carrying twins into a second trimester and feeling explosively, voluptuously, soppingly and insatiably sexy! Then you might also imagine my surprise when my usually sexually engaged partner found me, a mother-to-be, somewhat ... unsexy. Suffice to say that we experienced a number of missed opportunities.

Sadly, my post-delivery body did not feel as sexy as my pregnant body. The blissful and sleep deprived months that followed the delivery of our twins were filled with all modes of childcare and next to no sex. Who could think beyond the next feeding? I also think my partner found my lactating maternal breasts to be about as sexy as my previously pregnant body. My social circle, however, was quite taken by my expanded bra size. Public displays of tandem breastfeeding—necessary on a couple of occasions such as a holiday party couch feeding at a good friend's—garnered the close attention of our friends and acquaintances. I do not believe that these moments were interpreted as displays of sexuality; rather I was considered an oddity— a sort of "third sex"—similar to how I was treated when once on a diplomatic trip to Yemen. In this case, back in Toronto, my cow-like lactating breasts, overflowing from my sparkly metallic hot pink holiday top, signaled my "essential" duty: NOT partying with my friends. Thus, my maternal persona was big-breasted, soft and squishy but not in a sexual way. I believe that I started to internalize these reactions so that I did not feel particularly sexual, with or without the sexual attention. Professionally, I recall one film audition, about six months after giving birth, when I had lost a couple of dress sizes but was not back to my pre-pregnancy weight. There was lots of chatter and clucking (usual in the world of acting) between my agent and the casting director about how much weight I had lost and how good I looked. However, I did not get the job, and no matter how you cut it, being unemployed is not sexy.

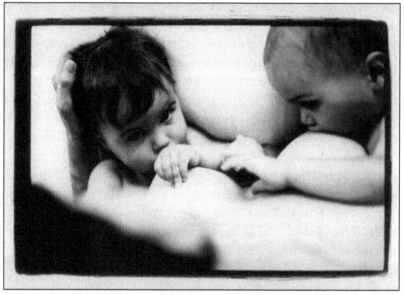

Figure Two. Mother (Terri) nursing babies (Alexa and Jake). Toronto. © 2001. Susan Maljan.

Here I must turn to sensuality, a feeling that was very present during my fifteen months of breastfeeding (Figure Two). I recall attending an educational investment group, a short-lived activity when my children were a few months old. One of the women in the group shared her view that breastfeeding her son was a much more sensual experience than breastfeeding her daughter. I kept that in mind, although I did not find the sensual relationships with my son and daughter to be gendered; rather, I found that the sensual connection ebbed and flowed at different times. Since I nursed my twins for fifteen months, and weaned them at the same time, I had my own "psych 101 experiment" at home. What I experienced was that my daughter was much more fixated on my breasts and nipples, and this fascination carried on well past the stage of weaning. She had no qualms about reaching down my shirt or looking for my breasts—just to touch or, perhaps, to make sure my nipples were still there. I recall that this continued until she was of kindergarten age. I even allowed her to suckle my nipples briefly a few times over those early years, although there was no milk to be had. She seemed to want the emotional and physical connection; instinctually, I responded. My son seemed to wean a bit more easily and did not show the same continued fascination with my breasts until, as a young child, he declared his intention to marry me. I noticed that his hugs and cuddles lingered a little longer and involved squishing against my chest or pushing off my torso and "accidentally" touching a breast or two. His was a curiosity that struck me as healthy, although I redirected his hands and shared the harsh reality that I was already married.

Thus, my experience with sensuality and sexuality has been that my pregnancy aroused hormones, feelings, and thoughts that might have made a sex therapist blush. When I was actively engaged in breastfeeding two children for ten to twenty hours a day, I had little interest in conjugal sex but felt sensual, fulfilled, and bodily charged through my tactile and emotional relationships with my children. In fact, my greater physical need was to *not* be touched— by anyone—for at least short periods of the day. Now that I am the mother of teens and have entered menopause, my feelings of sexuality require a bit more effort. A lack of hormones, ongoing fatigue, professional and academic responsibilities, and routinized lifestyle choices have likely contributed to a minimal decline in sexual activity. My experiences lead me to extend other theorists' observations of non-sexualized maternal breasts and argue for a right to sexualized or non-sexualized breasts at any time--whether they be maternal or non-maternal. The key, perhaps, is negotiating expectations with your partner (i.e., double rich chocolate or fat free sherbet?).

Flavour Three: Public and Private Pistachio
As I wrote in my MA Major Research Paper "The Millennial Wean,"

> Many of the (academic) readings of the last twenty-five years use history, economics and gender studies to seek to explain the division between the public and private spheres as they relate to breastfeeding. Most scholars also show that these socially constructed "spaces" (physical, emotional, and mental) and units of time affect breastfeeding theory and practice. In return, mention has been made of the influence choices in breastfeeding may have on reifying the social construction of these spheres. Some authors focus on essentialism as contributing to the creation of the public and private spheres (Blum; Hausman, *Mother's Milk*; LLL; Bartlett). Some extend the creation of the private sphere as a necessity for encompassing the health of the infant (LLL). Others cite the tensions between viewing breastfeeding as unpaid work as opposed to maternal obligation (Carter). Some scholars dwell on the social construction of the private sphere as related to decorum, womens' issues, and breastfeeding as a private practice (Carter; LLL). A few warn of the difficulties of breastfeeding and pumping breast milk in the public sphere (LLL; Bartlett; Stearns). We are told that issues of class, race, and privacy serve to blur boundaries between the public and private divide (Carter; Blum) and that public policy helps perpetuate the divide, supporting government goals around issues such as population growth. Some academics are concerned with a lack of feminist scholarship supporting breastfeeding choices (Hausman, *Mother's Milk*; Blum); others call for the contestation of social values which support these divisive public and private spheres (Bartlett), and some invoke mothers' bodies as one of the more dominant sites of contestation (Bartlett; Giles "Fountains," *Fresh Milk*). Some authors criticize the expectations of positive emotional engagement that seem to come with the creation and use of the private sphere (Friedman); still others look

beyond the public/private spheres to issues of survival for both mother and infant (Hausman, *Viral Mothers*). The vast majority of scholarly texts shine a critical light on the public/private divide, suggesting that the social construction of this division limits women's choices around infant feeding in the Global North. (48-50)

Personally, I wish that I had been more aware of these social issues at the time I was breastfeeding twins; I could have used my position in a more public way and joined the (l)activist movement of social resistance. As it was, I was an accidental activist, sometimes intervening in socially acceptable modes of behaviour largely out of necessity.

I have already shared my story of my holiday party public breastfeeding on display in the public sphere. I have also contrasted my accepted public work experience in one sound studio against a lost job in another studio because of the (projected) fears of the producer, and what I imagine was his aversion to "mixing" (industry pun intended) voice work with the work of mothering. Largely, I nursed our children at home—at our oversized breastfeeding station or in our townhouse's private courtyard. Thus, I intuitively chose the most convenient geographic location: the private sphere. I also recall the feedings of urgent necessity while we were in the public sphere—those moments when the babies were howling with hunger and would not wait. Sometimes, they would time these cries exquisitely—like when I happened to be in a coffee shop and could enjoy a vanilla steamed milk while allowing my babes to enjoy it second hand. In that café, I made a half-veiled attempt at discretion, never completely succeeding because of the logistics of feeding two babies at a time. At other times, I was caught off guard, such as one chilly November day, midway through a long walk in a park when one baby started to wail, shortly followed by the second. Although I ran, pushing the double carriage as fast as I could to make it to the sanctuary of our cozy home, I finally succumbed to the babies' calls for nourishment, lest they fade away in the remaining twenty minutes of travel. So I found myself sitting in an exposed field, nursing two babes, football-hold, breasts bared to the zero degree winds while a few bundled passersby tried not to stare at the unfortunate and ill-mannered mother squatting in the field, or so I imagined. At that moment, I definitely felt that I was performing a private act in a public place, although it was not the social stigma that was so unnerving; rather, it was the discomfort of the cold wind and the damp grass and the lack of a nursing pillow to support my aching back and shoulders. Perhaps there was something to this private sphere after all.

More telling than the times when I did breastfeed in public were the times when I chose not to. Sometimes, I chose not to take my babies with me to a public event or work engagement—just to avoid the logistical challenges and imagined censorship. I would spend hours pumping to give myself two extra hours of "away time" when we had a caregiver on hand, followed by hours of angst away from my children at an audition or recording gig—neither environment conducive to pumping—while my breasts filled up, tingling. I would rush home to find both babies in tears and their caregiver valiantly hopping around the living room, trying to comfort and bounce both babies simultaneously when the pumped milk I left was not enough. What would have been wrong with taking those babies (and the caregiver) with me to that particular workplace or appointment? In part, it did not seem professional to audition for the role of a thirty-something single (sexy) woman with two babies in tow. In part, I was self-conscious that I had hired a caregiver to care for my children because of my unpredictable and erratic work schedule, but mostly I was embarrassed because I could afford to pay for help and some of my friends could not. Thus, I was troubled by issues of the private and public spheres as well as class and privilege and was not aware enough or confident enough to contravene the normal patterns.

Perhaps my most memorable separation from my infants was on September 11, 2001, the tragic day of terrorist attacks on the United States. I had been hired to work that day; I was to act opposite Canadian icon Gordon Pinsent in a radio drama produced by the Canadian Broadcasting Corporation (CBC). As I was leaving my children in the capable hands of our caregiver Eva, I received a call from my longtime friend, journalist Donna Tranquada, urging me to turn on the television. I then drove to the CBC with the knowledge that one errant plane had "inadvertently" crashed into one of New York City's World Trade Center buildings. By the time I had reached CBC, two planes had crashed and the rest is history. I spent the day in the sound studio and took breaks to phone home to check on my children and to slip down to the CBC lobby to watch the news displayed on nine mega screens, my jaw glued to the floor. I scurried back to the studio, checked on my children, etc. My partner Jeff hurried home from his business at the Toronto International Film Festival (shut down for the first time in its history) to be with our children (bringing along several out of town friends); Eva rushed home to her son.

In retrospect, I must admit that Jeff was perfectly capable of caring for our children on this day. For my part, however, I hated being unable to be there for my kids. For some reason (which seems inexplicable in hindsight, but was probably a difficult decision for the producer at the time), the CBC crew continued to record this radio drama while the rest of Toronto's downtown core emptied out. I retain a searing mental image of having lunch with the lovely Gordon Pinsent at a hip restaurant on King Street and being the only customers in the joint, although the restaurant staff was seemingly trapped with us, too. Toronto was a ghost town. My children were home without me during what would become one of the most pivotal historical events in our lifetime. I could not go to them (without losing my job and letting down a team, I thought), and they could not come to me (nor perhaps would I have wanted them to), but we were definitely separated by the so-called public and private spheres. In this case, the private sphere seemed sheltered and safe. The public sphere seemed cold and scary—with an uncertainty of what might happen to this significant public building that I was working in—amid this incomprehensible cloud of attacks on public and private institutions. I was glad my children were home, yet I agonized that I could not be with them.

Yet, later, the greater agony was for the parents and children who had been caught in the four affected planes and in the World Trade Center—a workplace with excellent childcare facilities, a cutting-edge attempt at merging the public and private. In most cases, I would argue for this mixing up of spheres to create an overlapping Venn diagram of public and private. In this case, I was happy to have my children "safely" in the private sphere, unaware that "safety" was a concept now forever changed. Thus, in theory, although it sometimes seems more familiar and comforting to fall into the delineations of private and public, in practice it does not always work. Ultimately, I argue for mixing it up—supporting women in lactating, breastfeeding or bottle-feeding in public and supporting mothers or fathers who bring their children to the workplace along with a plan for success, which may include a support system of infant feeding equipment, space, and care-givers. I also advocate for parental choice—the choice to either bring children to the workplace or not; or the choice to provide infant feeding in a multitude of ways, in public or private, in a reasoned, responsible manner that supports the parents as well as the child. Each scenario requires awareness, education, and policies that support equal access to these solutions. This brings us back to the concept of the milkshake, a mixture of the public and private to be used every day or on infamous occasions such as 9/11. The key ingredients and amounts are to be determined by the primary caregiver(s), making every milkshake unique and, hopefully, delicious.

Flavour Four: Medicalized Marshmallows

One of the catchphrases of scholarship in maternal studies is the "medicalization of maternity and infant feeding." By this term, I mean that at some point the practice of infant feeding began to be treated as a medical problem. Academics have long questioned the place of women and children in the health industry over the last century or longer, specifically with regard to their treatments as a result of scientific "advancements". My central question in this realm is the following: has the medicalization of women and children affected the practice and theories of infant feeding, and if so, how?

As I noted in "The Millennial Wean,"

Most of the feminist scholars examined here cite the medicalization of breastfeeding as a mixed blessing. In reviewing the last two centuries of infant feeding prac-tices in the Global North, the death rate of women and children in the Global North has decreased, as the shift of power from midwives and mothers to doctors and medical experts has become apparent (Carter; Blum). The focus in infant feeding has primarily centred on the health of the child, though opinions as to what contributes to good infant health has shifted over time, leading to movement in public perception and subsequent adjustments in practices of infant feeding (Carter; Blum). Alongside the push for women's independence in the feminist movement, women's choices were influenced by scientific support advocating for the nutritional value of formula and the safety benefits of pasteurization, leading to greater use of bottle-feeding in the 1950s (Carter). Inequities around "choice" persisted among mothers, largely due to class and race; middle class mothers largely supported the medicalized movement. Public policy in health care veered towards the subsidization of formula in an attempt to level this playing field (Carter; Blum). Ultimately doctors and health practitioners were imbued with the status of "expert," and mothers relied less on their own embodied knowledge and instincts (Blum). Despite the well-meaning intentions of the medical community, a lack of informed choice persisted as a result of gaps in practical infant feeding knowledge and education (Carter; Blum; Giles, "Fountains," *Fresh Milk*). (66-67)

My extended experience with the medicalization of motherhood began with my efforts to have a successful pregnancy. As I alluded to earlier, having endured a number of miscarriages, I turned to medical practitioners and proceeded to involve myself in three years of tests, injections, and travels to Canadian and U.S. doctors with different theoretical bents. By the time I was into the second trimester of my only viable pregnancy, I was well acquainted with the medical system and grateful for the progress that my partner and I had made with its assistance. However, I always felt that I straddled the line between a blind acceptance of Western medicine and interventions and alternative medical practices, many of which relied on my intuition and self-knowledge. I opted for a combination of the two. I dutifully attended doctor appointments and a series of regular ultrasounds and poked my stomach and legs with needles every day to support the pregnancy while I simultaneously outlined a detailed and trendy holistic "birth plan" for our two babies and myself. My obstetrician/gynecologist—after patiently answering my three pages of questions at every appointment and fielding requests to avoid anesthesia when delivering the babies "naturally"—cautioned (and I'm slightly paraphrasing here),

> Terri, the next time you have a baby, I'll deliver it in a field, but this time, you're in a hospital. You're carrying twins. You will be in an operating room with full equipment, me, a resident doctor, an anesthesiologist, two pediatricians, nurses, and more. This is a HIGH RISK pregnancy. And no, you don't need to have a Caesarean section unless it's an emergency."

He stayed true to his word.

I did read every mainstream birthing book and bring every toy imaginable to the hospital for the delivery of our babies: yoga mat, yoga pillow, yoga bolster, a cooler of sandwiches, massage cream, raspberry leaf tea, meditation tapes, breathing tapes, and a real live doula. And yes, I did go through about twenty-four hours of labour. But after the first baby arrived vaginally ("Baby A" as the medical team dubbed her—later we named her Alexa), my doctor patiently waited while I put her on my chest and sang a song that I'd sung to her in utero for the last nine months.[3] The medical team then whisked my daughter away for her *Apgar* (medical) tests. (Although I "knew" she was perfect, I still asked my partner to follow and stay with her.) Back to the business of delivering baby number two, I pushed, and pushed, but he just was not budging. Finally, my doctor offered one last try before we resorted to a Caesarian section. I had a little confab with "Baby B" (later named Jake) and told him that I was not about to go through a vaginal delivery and a C-section in the same day. I asked him to push with me. He did. I did. With the aid of a set of medical forceps, our son emerged vaginally and unscathed. I also had the artsy option of singing a different vocal selection to him while he nestled on my chest.[4] We had two beautifully healthy babies (and two impressive placentas) and life was better than I ever could have imagined. And then I fainted.

Following the birth of our children, my doctor supported my extended stay at the hospital, and I had the opportunity to attend Women's College Breastfeeding Clinic. I also was given these few days to deal with a severe case of hives that had erupted over my entire body hours after giving birth—conveniently everywhere except my nipples. It was at that time that I appreciated the medicalization that we were exposed to, alongside my mother's dogged advocacy for her suffering daughter. After I had spent seventy-two hours sleeplessly wandering the hospital halls in an excruciating state of bodily itchiness, my mother pushed for a referral to a second dermatologist who recognized my rare condition as PUPPP, a post-pregnancy skin inflammation often linked to twins. I was prescribed prednisone for a period of seven weeks. After clearing this prescription with Mother Risk,[5] I concluded that this would be safe for my breastfeeding children, and I started the road to recovery and a blissful few hours of interrupted sleep per night. (That's right—there would be no uninterrupted sleep for years to come). For this medical intervention, I was extraordinarily grateful. In fact, the whole experience of being granted two healthy children six years after our first miscarriage was cause to thank and revere the medical community, despite a few ineffectual apples in the medical basket. I am still emotional at the thought of it. Six years after our first miscarriage, we were the parents of two healthy babies.

My experience of breastfeeding began in a medicalized environment. Prior to giving birth, I naively took for granted that I would breastfeed and was proactive in my planning with the Toronto Parents of Multiple Births Association. There I purchased used, oversized nursing pillows and baby clothes to prepare for a change in life that I could not yet fully comprehend. I received tips on how to nurse (or not nurse) and felt supported as I prepared to enter this daunting new world of parenthood. I assumed that I would breastfeed. Why? Because my mother had, and the medical and parenting literature supported that choice for the baby's health (Sears; Spock; Noble; Leach). Martha Sears (RN) and William Sears (MD), for example, argue that breastfeeding is the best and only choice, with the implication that their medical credentials positioned them as voices of authority (Sears and Sears 118-191).

The breastfeeding clinic in Women's College Hospital was extremely supportive in helping me navigate the difficult task of nursing two babies in tandem, and in answering my many questions about the different stages of the milk coming in, often referred to as "let down." I found it physically tough to manoeuvre two small beings on and off my body, and, initially, I found very little grace in doing so. However, my determination to give my children the "best" carried me through, and within days, I was capably breastfeeding. As our babies were somewhat small (4 lb. 14 oz. and 5 lb. 11 oz.), it was recommended by my medical team that I temporarily supplement their breast milk with formula, dispensed in the form of "finger feeding." This technique consisted of filling a syringe with baby formula and attaching it to a tiny tube taped to an adult's finger. The baby would suck on the finger and, simultaneously, draw formula from the tube. I was marginally concerned about the possibility of this interfering with the babies' desire for the breast, but mostly I was focused on their size, weight, and development. The brilliance of this form of feeding is that it allows other caregivers to engage in the infant feeding process in a very intimate and profoundly useful way. The image of my father and partner, finger feeding two babies in tandem, might be enough to convince anyone of the gaps in the argument of essentialism (Figure Three). If I had, in that moment, "popped off" from a bad case of hives, I have no doubt that my father and partner, with a little support from my mother and in-laws, would have raised our children beautifully without their "essential" mother. Thus, this medical intervention (which, in another time, might have been similar to advice dispensed by midwives) was integral to my children's' development and allowed me to work on my own production of milk and personal health in a way that was less pressured.

Through the excellent medical support of Women's College Hospital, and my own intuitive learning curve, I was able to navigate

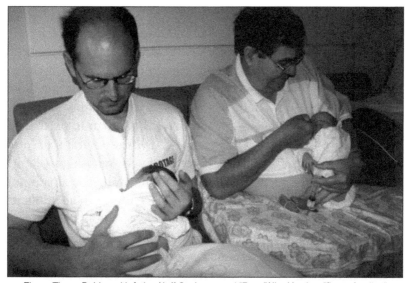

Figure Three. Babies with father/Jeff Sackman and "Papa"/Jim Hawkes "finger feeding" formula. Toronto. 2000. Grandma/Joanne Hawkes, photographer.

the pregnancy and the early months of infant feeding with success and confidence, although I know not everyone has such a fortuitous journey. Looking back, I would use my personal experience to support a hybridity of Western medical support and alternative practices. I do not believe that I would have two biological children today if it had not been for the medical advancements in Western medicine. I also may have suffered with excruciating hives for much longer without Western medicine, which no doubt would have greatly tested my mental health. Yet I also benefitted from alternative forms of medicine such as self-hypnosis, yoga, massage, and embodied practices, which prepared and supported me throughout this journey. I was the lucky beneficiary of all this, largely because I am fortunate enough to be positioned in Canada, a country with socialized medicine. I was privileged to have the necessary resources for private interventions with regard to my repeated miscarriages, and I am in a community that is aware of and supports the notion of alternative health practices. I was hugely fortunate to "have it all" and thus found no fault in combining these two streams of health support.

Instead of finding fault with the medical community and the "medicalization" of maternity, maternal feminists would do well to focus on increasing access to these as well as alternative streams of care and support. Every woman's journey is different: one may benefit from medical intervention, while another may not. With funding to support women in educating them around their choices and options and to create possible courses of action for those whose options are limited, we increase the possibility of better physical and mental health for mothers, children, and partners. I argue for a twenty-first-century goal of hybridity with regard to Western medical and alternative practices. Such a goal might require revision of government health policies to include social support for alternative intuitive health practitioners; workplace policies that prioritize infant feeding support; economic policies around daycare options for working-class families and mother-centred support groups (physical, mental, and emotional); and a shared knowledge exchange that ultimately reinforces social support for this two-streamed way of knowing.

Flavour Five: Goody, Goody Gumdrops

In "The Millennial Wean," I refer to the relatively new discipline of maternal studies, which some pinpoint as having gained traction in the 1980s:

> Adrienne Rich's thirty-year-old definition of "motherhood" as a patriarchal institution that has been culturally constructed by centuries of history[6] has evolved through a number of maternal theorists to define the last two decades as a period of extreme or "intensive mothering," defined by an unattainable standard of perfection – leading to labels such as the "good mother" (Hays; O'Reilly, "Introduction," *Mother Outlaws*). In defining the "good mother," maternal theorists of the last twenty years have explored the contradictions between selfless nurture and selfish ambition (Hays), unpaid and paid work tensions for union workers (Luxton) and "mother-actors" (Hawkes, "The Invisibility"), media representations of the ideal "New Momism" (Michaels and Douglas), debunking of myths of motherhood (Thurer), mother valorization versus mother-blame (Caplan), perils of "The Motherhood

Religion" (Warner), the false front of perfection known as the "mask of motherhood" (Maushart), "sensitive mothering" (Walkerdine and Lucey) and "natural" mothering, which Chris Bobel argues is paradoxical because it fails to acknowledge the privilege necessary to reclaim domesticity and maternity as a source of empowerment for women (Bobel). Andrea O'Reilly contends that "the current discourse of intensive mothering emerged in response to women's increased social and economic independence women would forever feel inadequate as mothers, and work and motherhood would be forever seen as in conflict and incompatible" (*Mother Outlaws* 10). These theorists all contribute to the prevailing view in women's studies that phrases such as "intensive mothering" or the "good mother" serve to disempower women in the western construct of patriarchal motherhood. I argue that the historical and current social construction of the "good mother" neatly parallels the social judgment of infant feeding; thus, a "good mother" in the Global North's new millennium is a "good breastfeeder" and must practice breastfeeding (preferably exclusively) for at least six months. In other words, the performance of breastfeeding, as dictated by medical decrees, social norms and expectations, and complicated by race, class, gender and sexuality, is inextricably intertwined with and helps determine a mother's cultural value. (70-71)

The previous examples of my determination to breastfeed my children lead me to conclude that my breastfeeding practice was consciously and unconsciously motivated by my desire to be a "good mother." Actually, many of the choices that I have made in my adult life were likely partly informed by parental and societal expectations that I be a "good daughter," "good student," "good employee," "good friend," "good sister," "good wife," and ultimately, a "good mother." Where does the definition come from? In retrospect, much of my construction of a "good mother" came from parenting literature, popular literature, and from a keen observation of parenting styles in my community. My desire to mother fully and completely was exacerbated by my six-year journey to give birth and the fact that giving birth to two babies at once completely rocked my world, making it impossible (and undesirable) to continue as I once had. Now my complete focus and energies were directed towards my two babies and their survival, then happiness, then development. It is only in retrospect that I can identify my goal to be a "good mother" as defined in the "Millennial Wean" kind of way. I completely bought into the new millennium middle-class requirements for intensive mothering. For me that meant performing a myriad of tasks: exclusively breastfeeding as long as possible, pumping as a last resort, feeding on demand, co-sleeping with babies, attachment parenting, reading to the babies from day one, playing classical music frequently, allowing only rare glimpses of educational television programs, only providing solid food that was organic and pureed, early enrollment in music classes and any educational and artsy opportunities I could find, creating tummy time, back time, mommy time, daddy time, grandparent time,[7] and all the trendy requirements of intensive mothering. But I didn't do it to be trendy. Intuitively, I loved creating all these educational and artistic opportunities, which is a practice that I continue today. On top of that, intellectually, the arguments around the benefits of breast feeding and organic purees made perfect sense to me. So what was the issue?

The issue, as I now see it, was that I learned to put my needs aside in my fervent desire to put my children's needs first. Such a decision was not unique or groundbreaking; it seems rather traditional and unimaginative, actually.[8] Yet I would likely do it again. Maybe I would spend more time getting my career back on track earlier in the parenting process, but if I could do that, *and* do the rest I would probably still do it. Although what felt "right" for me would not necessarily be healthy for another parent. I suggest that it is potentially problematic to categorize someone's choices as "good" and label a set of choices as "good parenting" or "good mothering," or whatever value-laden moniker is the trend of the moment. Popular parenting literature and practices often paint a picture of unattainable perfection and often lack an examination of issues of class, race, education, gender, sexuality, ability, and culture. I strongly object to current pop culture suggestions that an inevitable divide exists between mothers who work inside the home and those who pursue paid work outside the home; there is room here to develop a maternal community peppered with diverse models of parenting and a spirit of generosity. I argue that the solutions lie in increased education, awareness, and access. These key concepts present themselves in response to each of the aforementioned categories and emerge here again. As the feminist academic maternal literature has begun to question and examine the prerequisites of being a "good mother," so must popular literature and practice.

There is room for feminist writings in the arena of parenting literature and medical journals. The ultimate goal might be to support mothers, fathers, and other caregivers in their understanding of the social constructions of parenting and to provide them with a set of tools for determining what is best for their family, regardless of an arbitrary perception of what constitutes "good mothering" or "good parenting."[9] After increased awareness and education, the very real challenge remains in empowering all parents to gain access to increased support systems. Thus, although some current academic literature calls for regaining control of infant feeding and an examining of middle-class anxieties between mothers who work inside and outside the home, I would extend this call to include research around devalued and/or non-white-racialized caregivers, discomfort around breastfeeding in public, and political-economic policies designed to support low-income parents.

Thus, I argue for public advocacy for diversified practices of infant feeding, including (l)activism and alternative representations of lactating and/or non-lactating mothers in the arts, media, performance and other fields. A review of public policies, towards supporting a greater scope of mother's choices around infant feeding practices in public, in the workplace, or at home would be helpful. These goals could be enhanced by increased public and maternal education to support multiple choices of mothering practices. I also propose an exploration of the lack of scholarship around mothers with different abilities and how that may or may not affect their choices and options around infant feeding. All of these would go a long way towards mitigating the judgment that accompanies constructions like the "good mother."

Flavour Six: Sharing Sherbet

The sixth area that I have identified as integral to current academic discourse around infant feeding focuses on milk sharing. As recounted in "The Millennial Wean,"

Feminist historians (Carter; Blum; Hausman, *Mother's Milk*) retell the journey of the wet nursing and infant feeding practices in the U.K. and the U.S. From the seventeenth to the nineteenth centuries, paid wet nursing was the practice of choice for the aristocracy and financially independent artisans. In the late 1800s clinics emerged with opportunities for institutionalized wet nursing (Blum; Carter; Bromberg Bar-Yam), in an attempt to support working-class women who were not able to breastfeed. Increased medicalization and advances in knowledge and equipment led to more infant feeding options in the twentieth century. In response to war torn dwindling populations, many nations developed policies to support population growth (Carter; Blum; Nathoo and Ostry) and supported infant feeding through breast milk advocacy as well as bottle-feeding with newly developed formulas. There was some support for governmentally subsidized milk banks in the late nineteenth and early twentieth century, but that support and social demand dwindled by the mid-twentieth centuryy (Blum; Carter; Nathoo and Ostry). Informal milk sharing (Giles, *Fresh Milk*) is recorded in the twentieth century, with grass roots breastfeeding groups doing little to support this option (LLL). Most scholars report choices limited by any or all factors such as class, race, politics, science, technology, and socio-demographic forces (Carter; Blum; Hausman, *Mother's Milk*; Nathoo and Ostry). I would add to this list economics. The cost cutting trend for Canada's multi-layered governments at all levels makes new ventures challenging. Thus, the current government oversight and medicalization of breastfeeding and milk sharing contributes to a formal environment which seems to largely exclude formal wet nursing or milk sharing as a viable or affordable option. (93-94)

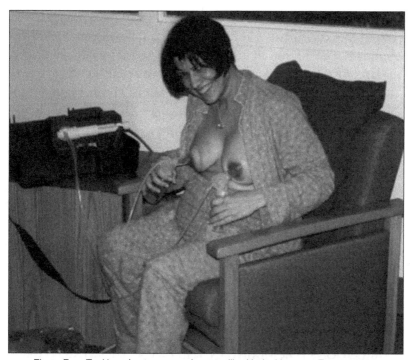

Figure Four. Terri learning to express breast milk with double pump. Toronto. 2000.
Joanne Hawkes, photographer.

Milk sharing is not something that affected me directly in my experience of infant feeding. I learned to pump at Women's College Hospital (Figure Four), temporarily equipped with their super double-barreled pump; I pumped often, although I rarely had extra milk to freeze. Sharing with others had not occurred to me, as I was preoccupied with making enough milk for two babies. However, a few superficial brushes with this practice helped expand my vision around what infant feeding could look like. Before I gave birth, I was at a café where I met a woman who was nursing her child. There she shared with me that she was an adoptive mother and was ingesting pills that induced her body to lactate, allowing her to breastfeed her child, although she supplemented the baby's diet with formula. This was new information to me, and when I was having difficulty carrying a child to term, I occasionally thought of this woman and the options that she had created for herself.

As an artist and academic who is interested in telling stories

of women's experiences and journeys, I have paid special attention of late to stories of infant feeding. I have not uncovered an
abundance of maternal infant feeding stories in the world of
theatre, film, and performance,[10] but those that do exist expand
our knowledge of what was and is possible in this realm (Ruhl;
Dobkin; Miller). My personal connection with milk sharing will
be "sharing milk stories," as I use my academic and autoethnographic research to weave a composite of infant feeding stories
in an effort to highlight women's experiences of mothering and
self-care. As there are gaps in academic and popular literature
around the subject of infant feeding, so, too, are there gaps in
theatre productions, performance art, and other performative
expressions of infant feeding and its attendant feminist discourse.
My form of (l)activism is a milk-saturated intervention into the
world of traditional, feminist, political, and activist theatre and
television. Stay tuned for my current theatrical work in progress:
Mother Knows Breast.

DIRECTIONS FOR MIXING IN THE TWENTY-FIRST CENTURY

The late-twentieth century and early twenty-first century was a
time that generated scholarship around breastfeeding, covering a
wide range of perspectives. In this chapter I have positioned my
Masters' research on academic theorizing of infant feeding between 1989 and 2013 ("The Millennial Wean"), and juxtaposed
these scholarly voices alongside my own personal experience and
knowing. In contextualizing my autoethnographic accounts of
breastfeeding between 2000 and 2001 within the larger subject of
infant feeding in the Global North, I touch on what I have identified
as six major subjects of current discourse in this field. Based on
my readings and my embodied experience of breastfeeding twins,
I argue for shared parenting practices and a strategic essentialism,
supported by awareness, education, and access to resources that
will support all parents in making choices that are most beneficial
for themselves, their children, and their families. Regarding the
sexualization of maternity, I call for a re-examination of sexualized
representations of lactating breasts in the creation of public performances (theatre, film, television, performance art and beyond).

Such a re-staging will, ultimately, make a contribution towards challenging heteronormative and gendered constructions of the great divide between sexuality and the maternal, which, by extension, will create space for alternative "performances" of breastfeeding—in theory, everyday practice, and creative representations of mothers. In examining social constructions of space, time and place (public and private spheres), I suggest there is value in a re-examination of breastfeeding and milk pumping practices in the public sphere, while also looking at the roles that class, race, and privacy may play in constructing these arbitrary spheres.

My own experience leads me to be curious about the impact of the "knowledge revolution" that has transformed workplace practices by relying on technology in a way that allows some parents to work from home. My home office-breastfeeding station physically combined my two major occupations, and I observe that this huge shift in the Global North has greatly affected parents' choices around childcare and infant feeding and should be considered as an important part of future scholarship in the area of infant feeding. Mixing up the social, cultural constructions and the practical considerations of motherhood as connected to infant feeding could help create a "milkshake" of overlapping spheres and infant feeding practices, supporting feminist scholarship around both breastfeeding and bottle-feeding, varied practices of infant feeding, and opportunities for cultural representations of alternative modes of blurred spheres of the private and public divides.

The belief that the medicalization of maternity has affected infant feeding theories and practices over the last century reveals a number of related threads of theory. I encourage continued dialogue around issues of class inequities, the freedoms of bottle-feeding, insufficient medical and social support to accompany the parallel medicalized and cultural demand for breastfeeding, imbalance of power between doctor or nurse and mother, and the knowledge-bridging properties of medical journals (Carter; Blum; Bartlett; Giles, *Fresh Milk*). My embodied experiences support an earlier position in which I called for a hybridity of medical and non-medical ways of knowing. I would be interested in seeing future research and subsequent shifts in public policy in maternal psychology as it relates to breastfeeding and other forms of infant feeding; a greater focus on maternal interests; maternal health and related issues around the subject of infant feeding; and the opportunity to bring unconventional, homeopathic and holistic ways of knowing into this discourse on medicalization. On a practical level, policy-makers could benefit from focusing on creating access to alternative health practices for all mothers and children.

I found my own infant-rearing practices and goals to be in accordance with the culturally constructed version of a "good mother," who practices breastfeeding for an acceptable period of time, selflessly nurtures, practices "natural" mothering, prioritizes the child, is usually white and affluent, follows medical expert pronouncements, shows "decent" conduct and responsibility, and bonds with her child(ren). In gaining retrospective awareness of my choices, I suggest now that there is clearly room for additional scholarship in examining infant feeding practices in relation to the constructions of "good" and "bad" mothers and the attendant complexities connected to race and class, employed and non-employed mothers, social mores around public breastfeeding, privacy and sexuality, and mothers with different abilities. Ultimately, the higher goal would be to determine if mothers are receiving adequate access to social, medical, and emotional support for the challenging choices and responsibilities they face as mothers, including their part in the responsibility of infant feeding. I have referred to the practice of milk sharing as a tool that could provide options for families that have difficulty accessing breast milk, which might contribute to enhanced choices for infant nutritional health and provide a rich source of material for further cultural projects. Although milk sharing is not directly connected to my personal embodied experience, the goal of "sharing milk stories" is. My milk sharing will emerge as part of my call to cultural producers to explore the complexities of breastfeeding and alternative forms of infant feeding, and the resonance these journeys have for maternal identities and health. Artists could consider exploring the fascinating world of milk gifting and commerce and the accompanying opportunities for dialogue around the practice of mothering, giving audiences a

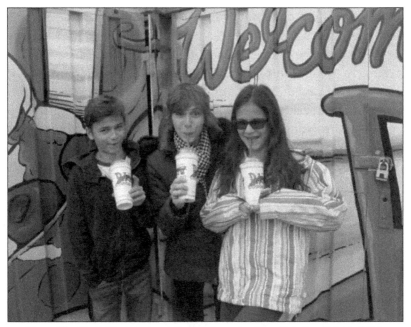

Figure Five. Terri with teenagers Jake and Alexa, slurping milkshakes. Calgary. 2013.
Photographer, Andrew Hawkes.

greater understanding of this complex yet simple practice, along-side other numerous opportunities for maternal storytelling.

MILKSHAKE SLURPING TECHNIQUE:
THE FLAVOUR IS IN THE MIX

My goal here has been to shed feminist light on twenty-five years of academic discourse around the subject of infant feeding as mediated by my autoethnographic accounts of breastfeeding in the new millennium. I have attempted to synthesize some of the louder voices in this dialogue, to re-situate research, to extend calls for future exploration, and to add my embodied perspective and voice to the mix—the milkshake mix, that is. In focusing on the Global North and the prevailing scholarly interest in essentialism, public and private spheres, sexualization of breasts, medicalization of maternity, construction of "the good mother," and milk sharing, I have attempted to create a landscape of the recent evolution and current position of infant feeding discourse. Concurrently, I have highlighted possibilities for future interventions in this field through research, public policy, everyday actions, and cultural productions. These interventions would honour both established scholarly thought alongside the wisdom of mothers and help to create a nuanced and tasty milkshake. Essential ingredients for a successful recipe must include a fluid blend of strategic essentialism, public and private overlapping spheres, expanded definitions of maternal sexuality, medicalized and alternative care partnerships, folded in with good and/or well-intentioned mothers—creating a powerful milkshake that shall be shared with others—theoretically, practically and culturally. This ideal formula would consist of equal parts awareness, education, and access. The flavour is in the mix. So indulge—mothers, fathers, caregivers and children (Figure Five); there are many more milkshakes to blend and slurp. Milkshake lovers, unite! *Serve with love.*

An earlier version of this paper was presented at the MIRCI conference "Mothers, Mothering and Motherhood from Ancient to Contemporary Times," Greece, 2014. I am appreciative of the conference participants' feedback. With regard to the theoretical components of this chapter, I acknowledge the wise guidance of my MA advisor, Andrea O'Reilly and second reader, Meg Luxton, and colleagues Lisa Sandlos and Paula John. Considering the practical components of this "early mothering" research, am indebted to Doctors Carl Laskin, Jon Barrett, Daniel Schacter and teams. I am thankful for my late mother Joanne Hawkes' passionate advocacy for my postpartum health; the loving presence of my father Jim Hawkes; the keen interest of my in-laws Mike (deceased) and Rhoda Sackman; the sterling maternal example of my late Grandma Amy Hartshorn; the kindnesses of co-caregiver Eva Almario; the treasured moral support of friends Clare Davenport, Donna Tranquada, Norma Dell'Agnese, Susan Cullen, Anne Campbell, and Jane Elliot; the superlative nighttime infant co-parenting of my partner, Jeff Sackman, and the incredible ongoing opportunities for growth with our beloved children, Alexa Hawkes-Sackman and Jake Hawkes-Sackman. I would also like to credit editor Kathy Mantas for embracing this merging of theory and practice. For all this, I am grateful.

NOTES

[1]Occasional reports of male lactation in times of stress or hormonal imbalance are cited throughout the literature examined here.

[2]Supporting the perspective that the work of mothering can be performed by persons of either gender, see Sara Ruddick and Andrea O'Reilly.

[3]I sang to my children in utero and after birth. One favourite was by Jule Styne, Betty Comden, and Adolph Green—"I Know a Place Where Dreams are Born" from *Peter Pan*.

[4]Our other favourite musical selection was by Jerry Bock, Joseph Stein, and Sheldon Harnick—"Sunrise, Sunset" from *Fiddler on the Roof*.

[5]"Mother Risk": A medical help line provided by The Hospital for Sick Children, Toronto.

[6]For further analysis of motherhood as an institution, see Adrienne Rich.

[7]My early interpretation of "good mothering" came from my own instincts, my observations of community practices and messages relayed in mainstream articles and parenting books such as cited below (LLL; Spock; Leach; Noble; Sears).

[8]For another perspective, see "Globe and Mail," citing an Atlantic study that child-centric parents derive more personal well-being from the parenting process.

[9]The scarcity or absence of the term "good father" perhaps reinforces social expectations of the mother as primary caregiver.

[10]For further analysis of the lack of mother-subjects in theatre, film, and performance art, see Hawkes "'Mother-Subjects' in Canadian Film: Off-Focus or Off-Screen?"

WORKS CITED

Bartlett, Alison. *Breastwork: Rethinking Breastfeeding*. Sydney: University of New South Wales Press Ltd., 2005. Print.

Blum, Linda M. *At the Breast: Ideologies of Breastfeeding and Motherhood in the Contemporary United States*. Boston: Beacon Press, 1999. Print.

Bobel, Chris. "Resisting, But Not Too Much: Interrogating the

Paradox of Natural Mothering." *Maternal Theory: Essential Readings*. Ed. Andrea O'Reilly. Toronto: Demeter Press, 2007. 782-791. Print.

Bromberg Bar-Yam, Naomi. "The Story of the Mothers' Milk Bank of New England." *Giving Breastmilk: Body Ethics and Contemporary Breastfeeding Practice*. Eds. Rhonda Shaw and Alison Bartlett. Toronto: Demeter Press, 2010. 98-109. Print.

Butler, Judith. *Gender Trouble: Feminism and the Subversion of Identity*. 1990. Preface. New York: Routledge Classics, 2010. Print.

Caplan, Paula J. "Don't Blame Mother: Then and Now." *Maternal Theory; Essential Readings*. Ed. Andrea O'Reilly. Toronto: Demeter Press, 2007. 592-600. Print.

Carter, Pam. *Feminism, Breasts and Breast-Feeding*. New York: Palgrave Macmillan, 1995. Print.

Dobkin, Jess. *The Lactation Station*. The Ontario College of Art and Design, Toronto. 2006. Performance.

Friedman, May. "For Whom Is Breast Best? Thoughts on Breast-feeding, Feminism and Ambivalence." *Journal of the Association for the Research on Mothering* 11.1 (2009): 26-35. Print.

Galupo, M. Paz and Jean F. Ayers. "Negotiating the Maternal and Sexual Breast: Narratives of Breastfeeding Mothers." *Journal of the Association for Research on Mothering* 4:1 (2002): 20-30. Print.

Giles, Fiona. "Fountains of Love and Loveliness: In Praise of the Dripping Wet Breast." *Journal of the Association for Research on Mothering* 4:1 (2002): 8-12. Print.

Giles, Fiona. *Fresh Milk: The Secret Life of Breasts*. New York: Simon & Shuster, 2003. Print.

Hausman, Bernice. *Mother's Milk: Breastfeeding Controversies in American Culture*. New York: Routledge, 2003. Print.

Hausman, Bernice. *Viral Mothers: Breastfeeding in the Age of HIV/AIDS*. Ann Arbor: University of Michigan Press, 2011. Print.

Hawkes, Terri. "'Mother-Subjects' in Canadian Film: Off-Focus or Off-Screen?" *Screening Motherhood in Contemporary World Cinema*. Ed. Asma Sayed. Toronto: Demeter Press, 2016. Print.

Hawkes, Terri. "The 'Millennial Wean': Performing Breastfeeding in the Global North—1989 to 2013." MA Major Research Paper.

York University, Toronto. 2013. Print.

Hawkes, Terri. "The Invisibility of Motherhood in Toronto Theatre: The Triple Threat." *Performing Motherhood*. Eds. Amber Kinser, Kryn Burton-Freehling, and Terri Hawkes. Toronto: Demeter Press. 2014. 247-269. Print.

Hays, Sharon. "Why Can't a Mother Be More Like a Businessman?" *Maternal Theory: Essential Readings*. Ed. Andrea O'Reilly. Toronto: Demeter Press, 2007. 408-430. Print.

Kinser, Amber. "Thinking About and Going About Mothering in the Third Wave." *Mothering in the Third Wave*. Ed. Amber Kinser. Toronto: Demeter Press, 2008. 1-16. Print.

Leach, Penelope. *Your Baby and Child*. New York: Alfred A. Knopf, Inc., 1997. Print.

La Leche League International. *The Womanly Art of Breastfeeding*, Seventh Revised Edition. New York: Plume/Penguin Group, 2004. Print.

Maushart, Susan. "The Mask of Motherhood." *Maternal Theory: Essential Readings*. Ed. Andrea O'Reilly. Toronto: Demeter Press, 2007. 460-481. Print.

Michaels, Meredith W. and Susan J. Douglas. "The New Momism." *Maternal Theory: Essential Readings*. Ed. Andrea O'Reilly. Toronto: Demeter Press, 2007. 617-639. Print.

The Milk Truck. By Jill Miller. Toronto, 2013. Performance.

Noble, Elizabeth. *Having Twins*. Boston: Houghton Mifflin Company, 1991. Print.

Nathoo, Tasnim, and Aleck Ostry. "Wet-Nursing, Milk Banks, and Black Markets: The Political Economy of Giving Breast Milk in Canada in the 20th and 21st Century." *Giving Breastmilk: Body Ethics and Contemporary Breastfeeding Practice*. Eds. Alison Bartlett and Rhonda Shaw. Toronto: Demeter Press. 2010. Print.

O'Reilly, Andrea. "Introduction." *Mother Outlaws: Theories and Practices of Empowered Mothering*. Ed. Andrea O'Reilly. Toronto: Women's Press, Canadian Scholar's Press, 2004. Print.

O'Reilly, Andrea. "Introduction." *Twenty-first-Century Motherhood: Experience, Identity, Policy, Agency*. Ed. Andrea O'Reilly. New York: Columbia University Press. 2010. 1-21. Print.

Rich, Adrienne. *Of Woman Born: Motherhood as Experience and Institution*. New York: W.W. Norton and Company, 1976. Print.

Ruddick, Sara. *Maternal Thinking*. Boston: Beacon Press. 1995. Print.

Ruhl, Sarah. *In the Next Room, or The Vibrator Play*. Berkeley Repertory Theater, 2009. Performance.

Sears, Martha, and William Sears. *The Breastfeeding Book*. Boston, New York and London: Little, Brown and Company, 2000. Print.

Shaw, Rhonda, and Alison Bartlett, Eds. *Giving Breastmilk: Body Ethics and Contemporary Breastfeeding Practice*. Toronto: Demeter Press, 2010. Print.

Smith, Paige Hall, Bernice L. Hausman, and Miriam Labbok, Eds. *Beyond Health, Beyond Choice: Breastfeeding Constraints and Realities*. New Brunswick, NJ: Rutgers University Press, 2012. Print.

Spock, Benjamin, and Steven Parker. *Dr. Spock's Baby and Child Care*. Revised and updated 7th edition. USA: Dutton/Penguin Group, 1998. Print.

Stearns, Cindy. "The Breast Pump." *Giving Breastmilk: Body Ethics and Contemporary Breastfeeding Practice*. Eds. Rhonda Shaw and Alison Bartlett. Toronto: Demeter Press, 2010. 11-23. Print.

Thurer, Shari L. "The Myths of Motherhood." *Maternal Theory: Essential Readings*. Ed. Andrea O'Reilly. Toronto: Demeter Press, 2007. 331-344. Print.

Van Esterik, Penny. *Beyond the Breast Bottle Controversy*. New Brunswick, NJ: Rutgers University Press, 1989. Print.

Van Esterik, Penny. "Breastfeeding and HIV/AIDS; Critical Gaps and Dangerous Intersections." *Giving Breastmilk: Body Ethics and Contemporary Breastfeeding Practice*. Eds. Rhonda Shaw and Alison Bartlett. Toronto: Demeter Press, 2010. 151-162. Print.

Walkerdine, Valerie, and Helen Lucey. "It's Only Natural." *Maternal Theory: Essential Readings*. Ed. Andrea O'Reilly. Toronto: Demeter Press. 224-236. Print.

Warner, Judith. "The Motherhood Religion." *Maternal Theory: Essential Readings*. Ed. Andrea O'Reilly. Toronto: Demeter Press, 2007. 705-725. Print.

White, Burton L. *The First Three Years of Life*. New York: Fireside, 1985. Print.

15.
Embryonic Motherhood

Interrogating the Rhetoric of Infertility, Assisted Reproductive Technology, and Mothers of Multiples in Tabloid Culture

MARIA NOVOTNY

A number of risks are associated with the use of illegal drugs during pregnancy including low birth weight, cerebral palsy, mental retardation, and respiratory problems. As a society, we condemn women who *knowingly* and *voluntarily* expose their would-be children to these risks. But what about the woman who finds out after months of painful infertility shots, months of monitoring her cycle, and years of trying to get pregnant, she finally succeeds? What if she discovers she is not just pregnant, but pregnant with seven fetuses? By choosing to try to carry all seven fetuses to term, this woman also *knowingly* and *voluntarily* exposes her would-be children to risks including low birth weight, cerebral palsy, and respiratory problems. Do we, as a society, treat this woman the same way we treat the woman who uses illegal drugs? The fact is we do not. (Shivas and Charles 183)

THIS ESSAY EXAMINES the complex rhetoric of mothering multiples and its impact on infertile couples contemplating the use of assisted reproductive technology (ART) treatments, such as in vitro fertilization (IVF). Currently, one in eight couples in the United States encounters difficulty in getting (and remaining) pregnant (CDC, "Reproduction Health"). In an attempt to build their families, many of these couples seek ART treatments, with approximately 85 to 90 percent of all infertility cases being treated with drug therapy or surgical procedures (Resolve, "Fast

Facts about Infertility"). In fact, data collected between 2006 and 2010 by the Centers for Disease Control and Prevention (CDC) reports that nearly 7.4 million infertile women have sought fertility services (CDC, "FastStats: Infertility"). For many heteronormative Western[1] infertile women, infertility is commonly associated with a failure to conform to cultural expectations of what it means to be a woman (Marsh and Ronner). Encountering an infertility diagnosis reorients individuals not only to their bodies but to the Western world's privileging of naturally conceiving and carrying one's own child. Evidence of the numerous reorientations one undergoes upon receiving an infertility diagnosis appears frequently in the navigation of multiple scenes in which the topic of infertility asserts itself:

> Infertility has been variously described as a syndrome of multiple origin, a consequence or manifestation of disease rather than a disease entity itself, a biological impairment, a psychosomatic disorder, a condition characterizing a couple rather than an individual, a failure to conform to cultural prescriptions to reproduce, and a failure to fulfill the personal desire to beget a child. (Sandelowski 477)

Sociologist and infertility scholar Arthur Greil finds that Western infertile women respond actively and strategically to their infertility diagnosis, frequently turning to fertility treatment to resolve their childlessness. With technological advancements for reproduction, especially with the creation of in vitro fertilization, cultural attitudes towards infertility suggest that it is not only a medical condition but one that is capable of being 'cured' through fertility treatment. In fact, Margarete Sandelowski and Sheryl de Lacey have noted the inventive nature of the concept of *in*-fertility:

> Infertility was "invented" with the in vitro conception and birth in 1978 of Baby Louise. That is, in the spirit and language of the Foucaudian-inspired "genealogical method"... infertility was discovered—or, more precisely, discursively created ... —when *in*-fertility became possible. Whereas barrenness used to connote a divine curse of

biblical proportions and *sterility* an absolutely irreversible physical condition, infertility connects a medically and socially liminal state in which affected persons hover between reproductive inability and capacity: that is, "not yet pregnant"...but ever hopeful of achieving pregnancy and having a baby to take home. (34-35)

Reproductive technologies, such as IVF, have thus affected the medicalization of infertility and risk of conceiving multiples. While medical advances with IVF have reduced the number of multiple births associated with IVF (Kulkarni et al.), there remains a 24 percent risk for multiples in ART-related pregnancies (Murray and Norman 222). According to the CDC, over one percent of all infants born in the U.S. are conceived through ART (CDC, "FastStats: Infertility"). Infertility's reliance on ART and ART's multiple birth rate reveal an increased chance for an infertile couple to conceive multiples. This essay examines the role of Western tabloid depictions of mothers with multiples from the lens of infertility and the increasing number of women relying on embryonic assistance to become mothers. While ART is often hailed as a technology to resolve infertile women's desire to experience pregnancy and motherhood (Sandelowski), tabloid culture portrayals of infertile mothering multiples are often scandalized. Surveying recent tabloid culture portrayals of mothering multiples in relation to infertility and the assumed risk of becoming pregnant with multiples through ART, this essay seeks to interrogate the intersections of infertility, reproductive technology treatments, and mothering multiples.

My interest in exploring the intersections of infertility and multiples developed out of prior conversations with other infertile women. Facing my own diagnosis of infertility, I frequently hypothesized with other infertile women about the possibility of conceiving and mothering multiples. Whenever the topic was broached, my mind would immediately pull up images of women with bursting pregnant bellies confined to bed rest. Often these images included tabloid depictions of mothers of multiples like Kate Gosselin, featured on the TLC reality series *Jon & Kate Plus 8*, or Nadya Suleman, often referred to in pop culture as the "Octomom" and featured several times on *The Oprah Winfrey Show*. While these images also frequented the minds of my infertile friends, I was struck by their openness and even willingness to embrace the idea of multiples. Transferring more embryos can be perceived as an attractive option, increasing one's likelihood to become pregnant. Yet increasing the number of embryos transferred can also increase one's risk to conceive multiples. Such conversations fueled my interest in exploring the politics of conceiving and mothering multiples because of infertility. I thus root my discussion of multiples around the topic of infertility in this essay.

FOUCAULDIAN BIOPOWER, INFERTILITY, AND MULTIPLES

To understand the rhetorical intersections of multiples and infertility, Foucault's concept of "biopower" serves as a theoretical frame to articulate how bodies, especially female bodies, are mediated through technology. In their introduction to *Body Talk: Rhetoric, Technology, Reproduction*, Lay et al. explore how the discourse of reproductive technologies shaped and continues to influence Western expectations of the female body. These advances in reproductive technologies arrived in part through what Foucault names as biopower, a concept derived from the need for managing population during the eighteenth century. That is, as Western nations began to derive more power and influence over the world, technologies to control and manage the births, deaths, reproduction, and illnesses of populations began to appear. This desire for nations to have power over the bodies of their constituents led to "an explosion of numerous and diverse techniques for achieving the subjugation of bodies and the control of populations" (Foucault 140), referred to as biopower.

Technological advances to control, monitor, and make more efficient the human body not only shaped the practices of individual bodies but also began to control larger societal and cultural ideologies about bodies. That is, while biopower has influence over individual subjects, it also influences larger cultural norms about the body. Often, these cultural norms and ideologies are articulated through authoritative systems of knowledge (science and/or medicine) and the display of power and authoritative discourse. In this way, how individuals viewed their bodies became highly mediated through authoritative knowledge systems, power, and discourses to control the body as desired by larger nation-state entities. Laura Mamo explains Foucault's theory on the regulation of bodies writing:

> Bodies and their subjectivities and identifications are constituted in and through relations of power-knowledge. The classifications of "infertility" and "homosexuality," for example, do not arise in nature, but are constituted by social and cultural systems of meaning, codified in cultural rules that define what is normal and abnormal. (9)

Questions regarding how to best treat and approach discussions of the body become expressed then through authoritative knowledges and discourses that support biopower's objective to control, monitor, and make efficient the human body. What thus emerged through biopower was a "normalizing" power—using authority, power, and discourse to articulate control over the action of bodies and distinguish functions of bodies as either "normal" or "abnormal." Biopower as a normalizing concept continues to be relevant to current issues of health, especially female reproduction.

Today, medical discourse continues to construct normalizing versions of the body. Biopower's relationship with authoritative knowledge systems remains extremely relevant given the numerous reproductive technologies developed to "fix" the female body. Infertility's dependence on ART is one such example. Elizabeth Britt has written about states passing infertility laws mandating individual states to cover reproductive technology treatment to infertile individuals. Such a law authorizes medical experts and the field of medicine as the legitimate solution to the issue of infertility. Specifically, Britt argues, "medical treatment for infertility has normalized the [infertile] experience" (208). The normalizing of infertility as a medical condition works to equate infertility with medical treatment by "providing symbolic and economic encouragement for women and couples to pursue this avenue of resolution to the often life-altering experience of infertility" (Britt 208). Britt's application of Foucault's concept of biopower to the experience of infertility expands the disciplinary role of medical discourse to categorize and diagnosis "normal" and "abnormal" bodies. That is, the infertile body from a biopower perspective is abnormal in that it fails to support human (re)productivity within an industrialized, capitalist society. Furthermore, the encouragement for infertile bodies to pursue reproductive technology treatment as a way to normalize the infertile body operates as a biopower construct. Reproductive technology treatment thus becomes the solution to "fix" the disease of infertility and the infertile body's inability to conform to capitalist society.

Biopower's influence on the experience of infertility—as needing to turn to reproductive technology treatments to fix the infertile body—resolves the "abnormal" body and adheres to cultural norms of having a family. Not only do reproductive technologies work to normalize the infertile body by creating alternative avenues for the infertile couple to conceive, but reproductive technologies also work to uphold cultural ideologies that privilege the family as the "best," "most appropriate," and thus "most desired" lifestyle. This reported desire to have a child and experience motherhood-parenthood frequently appears in contemporary medical literature on infertility (Greil, Slauson-Blevins, and McQuillan).

Yet medical literature is not the only place where such a desire to experience motherhood for infertile women through reproductive technologies is expressed. This narrative of infertile women desperately wanting motherhood continues to be told by social science scholars examining popular media outlets, like tabloid journalism, which describe "these technologies as beneficial—even desirable—to potential clients" (Diepenbrock 99). Women's magazines, public and social media outlets, and even reality television continually are saturated within biopower's normalizing discourse, motivating infertile women to resolve their abnormality through reproductive technology treatment.

Reproductive technology serves, then, to normalize the infertile body not only by resolving the infertile body's physical inability to conceive but by allowing that body to achieve a family and, more importantly, adhere to cultural norms and ideologies. Yet the risk attached to conceiving (and, in turn, mothering) multiples when utilizing reproductive technology challenges the normalizing effect of ART. Public discourses of motherhood privilege the reproductive technology story that provides the childless, infertile couple with one healthy baby—conforming to biopower's objective in yielding a "normal" Westernized orientation to pregnancy and parenting. Reproductive technology that results in the birth of multiples is frequently portrayed in public discourses as either obscure, scandalizing, irresponsible, or a burden to the general public, while the mother and medical doctor that approved the use of ART are usually shamed.

To understand the contradictions embedded within the public discourse of mothering multiples, I focus on public portrayals and public reactions to mothering multiples. Specifically, I describe public reception towards mothering multiples through the examples of "Octomom" Nadya Suleman, Kate Gosselin, and the more personal-interest story of Ashley and Tyson Gardner's reaction to learning that they conceived quadruplets, which was featured on the *Today Show*. An important element in selecting these examples is that all three women had identified as infertile and became pregnant through reproductive technology treatment. Furthermore, each example demonstrates three different reactions to the discourse surrounding multiples and leads to critical questions about how tabloid culture creates narratives of multiple births that often contradict one another and fail to expose the true health and medical risks involved in birthing multiples. In the end, questions are considered about the relationship between biopower's normalizing discourse and Western tabloid fascination with mothers of multiples.

NADYA SULEMAN

In January 2009, news broke that a woman living in California had given birth to octuplets. Initially, public reaction to this announcement was overwhelmingly positive. Yet two weeks later, as the public began to learn the identity of this single and unemployed woman, public opinion shifted drastically (Celizic). The woman, thirty-three year old Nadya Suleman, soon found herself on network television defending her decision to keep the octuplets, in addition to the six previous children she had conceived through reproductive technology and was currently raising. On television, she defended not only her decision to keep the children but her delight in the prospect of having such a large family. Public fascination with the logic Suleman employed to justify how she was providing for her children through unconditional love, yet no income, swept across the U.S. She made frequent appearances on *The Oprah Winfery Show* and received financial coaching from proclaimed finance guru Suze Orman. As publicity about the "Octomom" increased, the public criticized Suleman's desire for multiples. The adverse reaction to Suleman and to her reproductive endocrinologist, who knowingly implanted several embryos in an unemployed woman with the potential for conceiving multiples, led to the physician losing his medical license in 2011. While threats to remove the children from Suleman's home persisted, claiming she was an unfit mother raising a family of fourteen on welfare, Suleman continued to keep the children. She accepted a range of employment offers, from starring in the adult film *Octomom Home Alone* to partic-ipating in an online debate on parenting with Michael Lohan, father of Lindsey Lohan. Through these efforts and reliance on her newly found celebrity status as "Octomom," Suleman continues to raise all fourteen children.

KATE GOSSELIN

Kate Gosselin first introduced herself to the world in 2006 as a married mother of twins and sextuplets on the one-hour television special *Surviving Sextuplets and Twins*. This special focused on the difficulty Jon and Kate Gosselin faced in attempting to get pregnant because of Kate's polycystic ovarian syndrome diagnosis. The special documented how, through fertility treatments, Jon and Kate became pregnant with sextuplets and the day-to-day reality of mothering two sets of multiples. A major focus of the special was the management of the family's routine, which was displayed on various lists and charts throughout the house. In the special, Kate explains that while some may feel her management of the family is overboard, having a detailed routine in place helps her survive the task of raising two sets of multiples. Fascination with Kate's strict routine and mothering style captured the public's attention and the television series was soon followed up with a

Surviving Sextuplets and Twins: One Year Later special and an eventual recurring series titled *Jon & Kate Plus 8*. The airing of the *Surviving Sextuplets and Twins: One Year Later* special not only provided an update on the two sets of multiples but detailed how the airing of *Surviving Sextuplets and Twins* created avenues of support for Kate and Jon. Volunteers came over to assist with the day-to-day management of the household so that Kate could spend more time with the children and a local plastic surgeon even offered, knowing they could never afford the procedure, to provide a free tummy tuck on Kate. Viewers expressed sympathy towards Jon and Kate who openly talked about their financial struggles, tensions in their marriage, and how their Christian faith kept their family together. Yet, as the series *Jon & Kate Plus 8* aired over a period of two years featuring five seasons, the series came to a close as Jon and Kate announced their separation and eventual divorce.

Fans of the show rushed to Kate's defense as rumors surfaced of Jon's alleged infidelity. Yet critics of the show, who noted the repeated controlling aggression of Kate's parenting, began to erode some of the sympathetic support viewers held for Kate. While TLC aired the television series *Kate Plus 8*, detailing the life of Kate now as a single mother raising the sextuplets and twins, the show was ultimately put on hold; John threatened legal action and accused Kate of exploiting their children for profit.

Tabloids and public discourse around Kate Gosselin became much more critical of not only her parenting choices but physical evolution—accusing her of spending money from the show on her expensive clothes and plastic surgery. The image of Kate now as a reality-hungry mother desperately relying on reality television to support her family came to a head in early 2014 when she appeared on the *Today Show* with her twins, Mady and Cara. When asked by Savannah Guthrie of the *Today Show* about how their family was doing, both girls remained silent. Not knowing how to respond, Mady finally replied with the awkward "um," to which Kate quickly stepped in and scolded "Mady, your words—it's your chance, spit it out" (Pawlowski, "Gosselin Girls"). After such an awkward appearance, gossip magazines and talk shows were quick to critique Kate again as a controlling, humiliating mother. Kate Gosselin is an important example in understanding the complex rhetoric of mothering multiples, particularly in how public reception of her has shifted over the years. That is, the public starts out watching Kate recount her deep desire to have family and how the ability to undergo reproductive technology was a blessing that allowed her to have children. In the beginning, Kate is portrayed as a symbol of do-it-all motherhood and a pinnacle for Christian family values. Yet this image solely comes undone. She is no longer herald as a success story. Instead, with the unraveling of her marriage and the stress of raising a set of twins and multiples, Kate's image shifts to that of a controlling, humiliating, and aggressive mother of multiples. Reflecting on how Kate's narrative as a mother of multiples has shifted is important in pondering how identities of mothers can shift through public perception and discourse.

THEY'RE HAVING ... QUADRUPLETS:
ASHLEY AND TYSON GARDNER'S VIRAL PHOTOS

Public reactions to multiples have not been limited to only reality television. In the era of social media, reactions to conceiving multiples are frequently shared. For example, in early October 2014, photos capturing the shocked expressions of Ashley and Tyson Gardner quickly circulated on social media. One photo captured by a photographer during Ashley's ultrasound portrays her emotional reaction to the eye-popping news of successfully conceiving not just one baby—but four. Another photo shows the jaw-dropping faces of the couple staring at the camera in disbelief as they each hold two ultrasound photos (Samakow). After struggling for eight years to conceive because of infertility, the couple's reaction to discovering that Ashley was not only pregnant but carrying four fetuses trended on numerous social media and tabloid news outlets. The couple's reaction was featured on the nationally syndicated *Today Show* broadcast, in which the anchors described the viral photos as capturing a "priceless reaction" for the couple who "got the shock of the lifetime." As *Today Show* anchor Tamron Hall announced that they were having four babies, the three other anchors all cheered "it's perfect" and "we wish them the best" (Pawlowski, "After Eight Years").

As Ashley and Tyson's photos continued to circulate both on television and on social media outlets, the couple felt blessed for now having the opportunity to have the large family that they had always hoped for, noting the expense of having just one baby using IVF. Important to the story of Ashley and Tyson is that their reaction to having multiples not only intrigued the public but won its support and happiness—as seen through the *Today Show* excerpt. While other news and tabloid outlets critiqued mothers of multiples, like Suleman and Gosselin, these same outlets portrayed the viral photos of Ashley and Tyson as a couple trying to raise awareness around infertility by highlighting the realities of IVF cost and the emotional struggle of infertility when trying to create a family. The contrast of the public's reaction to Ashley and Tyson's announcement of multiples to that of Suleman's and Gosselin's mothering of multiples leaves questions about tabloid's culture influence over the rhetoric of multiples.

TABLOID CULTURE

The three examples describing public reaction to mothers of multiples are all situated in Anita Biressi and Heather Nunn's definition of tabloid media, which refers to journalistic practices that "prioritize entertainment, human interest and commercial profitability" (7). Linda Layne in her case study on Karen Santorum and Michelle Duggar, two women who publically documented their experience of pregnancy loss, uses the concept of "tabloid culture" to suggest how public expressions of pregnancy loss were often received by much negativity and criticism. Drawing on Freud's concepts of the "canny" and the "uncanny," Layne's theoretical framework is useful to examine the relationship between "tabloid culture," the canny, and the uncanny as it pertains to Suleman, Gosselin, and Gardner as public figures of mothers of multiples.

Henrik Ornebring and Anna Maria Jonsson explain that tabloid journalism "thrives on sensation and scandal" (23). Layne has thus argued that tabloid culture often sensationalizes what Freud describes as the uncanny. "The uncanny," according to Freud, is "unhomey, unfamiliar" and often experienced as "eerie, creepy, and weird," whereas "the canny" refers to that which is intimate, "concealed from sight" and evokes a sense of belonging to either the home or family. The canny then provides a sense of pleasure and security. Tabloid journalism often thrives on the uncanny by exposing intimate secrets of the home and/or family to the world. Suleman, Gosselin, and Gardner all exposed their intimate experiences with infertility to the world through the images of their multiples. In many ways, their openness about their inability to conceive situates all three of the women as uncanny. Their "uncanniness" is further amplified through their conceiving of multiples. Yet there are various layers to each individual's uncanniness, resulting in different degrees of sensationalism and varying reactions to the public images of these women as mothers of multiples.

Suleman is perhaps the most uncanny of the three. Almost immediately, her story became highly sensationalized, and she was often portrayed as a threat both to her home and to her children. As a single, unemployed mother of octuplets and other multiples, Suleman's character aligns to that of the uncanny—as weird and incapable of providing any security in the lives of her children. This level of uncanniness has resulted in a public outcry, charging Suleman as an unfit mother and even threatening to take her children away from her. This uncanniness is immediately represented, though, by her position as a single mother desiring a large family, with no secure income. While Suleman's story is rare, her uncanniness appears to be a condition of her non-conformance to traditional, heteronormative ideals. As a single mother of several children, conceived through fertility treatments, Suleman represents a new version of the welfare mother. Her desire to have a large family while being single and infertile raises questions about who are deemed appropriate users of ART to conceive. She threatens traditional images of mothers. For Suleman, reproductive technologies embedded within biopower have failed to provide a normalizing effect around the rhetoric of multiples for her because of her extreme uncanniness.

The example of Kate Gosselin, however, demonstrates how her openness about her infertility and use of fertility treatments were initially welcomed and supported by public viewers. While Gosselin was open about the private struggle to conceive, she constructed the story with her husband around topics of Christianity and marriage.

In this way, her story balanced the uncanniness of giving birth to multiples. Yet as her marriage eroded and she emerged as a more aggressive, masculine character, she took on an enhanced uncanny persona. As her uncanniness increased around speculations that she was a "mean mother" and that she exploited her children for her own personal success, tabloid culture began to rely on her uncanniness and began to create Gosselin as the "psycho-mom." Gosselin represents the degrees to which the uncanny can become revealed and how often the uncanny is presented as that which opposes traditional roles. The more Gosselin revealed a stricter, aggressive, masculine approach to her mothering, the more sensational of a character she became. Her increased sensationalism led to more public critique about her ability to mother multiples, especially as a now single mother. The depiction of Gosselin as a single mother attempting to provide for her sets of multiples through reality television and other publicity deals such as book deals and guest appearances challenges traditional roles expected of mothers, especially mothers who spent years trying to conceive in order to have family.

Ashley Gardner represents the more moderate version of the uncanny. While Gardner made the decision to expose her eight-year long struggle with infertility by blogging about her journey with various fertility treatments—bringing "out of the secret confines of the intimate home (and hospital life), into public view" (Layne 223)—she did so through practices that did not directly challenge or threaten traditional roles of mothering. Her story was documented as a journey she took not by herself but with her husband. Details about the financial sacrifices they made in order to save and pay the costs for IVF constructed an image: not only were they serious about wanting to have a family but they were financially responsible as well. Thus, while images of her reaction to having quadruplets went viral, public reaction to Gardner's response was well received, such as on the *Today Show* when all the anchors sent well wishes to the couple. Furthermore, the reaction of Gardner to the multiples aligns with a more "canny-like" response. Reacting with shock and qualifying the news as a "blessing," the Gardners adhere to more traditional, expected, and familiar reactions to news of multiples. Unlike Suleman and Gosselin, who both have become caricatures of mothers with multiples, Gardner's "un-canniness" is described only through her "bravery" to share her infertility journey. Her uncanniness does not become scandalized to the degree of Suleman and Gosselin, because Gardner adheres to expected, familiar, and traditional roles of an expectant mother.

FEMINIST CRITIQUES OF THE UNCANNY

What is learned then from these three representations of the un-canny mothering of multiples? In 2006, Andrea O'Reilly coined the term "motherhood studies," which articulates a distinction between "motherhood" and "mothering." According to O'Reil-ly, motherhood "is used to signify the patriarchal institution of motherhood" opposed to mothering, which "refers to women's lived experiences of childrearing as they both conform to and/or resist the patriarchal institution of motherhood and its oppressive ideology" (2). The patriarchal institution of motherhood confines the definition of mother "to heterosexual women who have bio-logical children" and further restricts the ideological concept of a good mother to "a select group of women who are white, het-erosexual, middle-class, able-bodied, married, thirty-something, in a nuclear family with usually one to two children, and ideally, full-time mothers" (O'Reilly 7). Feminists have sought to expand this limited construction of motherhood and the characteristics that define a good mother.

The uncanny mothering practices of Suleman, Gosselin, and even Gardner provide examples of how they challenge the patriarchal construction of motherhood. While Gardner most closely conforms to institutional expectations of motherhood, all three women as mothers of multiples clearly reject traditional characteristics of good mothers. Their choice to publically expose both their chil-dren and the medical processes they underwent to become parents threatens public perceptions of what is familiar. Freud cautions that the uncanny "is the class of the terrifying which leads back to something long known to us, once very familiar" (123-124). By being so open and available through tabloid journalism, the initial perception of having multiples as strange becomes less strange and more familiar as these mothering practices are made more visible.

While tabloid journalism attempts to capitalize on the uncanny portrayals of mothering—seen through Suleman, Gosselin and Gardner—what fails to be realized is that through this constant exposure, public perception of mothering multiples is made less obscure, less sensationalized. In fact, the concept of mothering multiples in the infertility community has become more welcomed because it can be financially savvy and can fulfill a deep desire for these women to have a biological family of their own (Reddy). In this way, the rhetoric of mothering multiples within tabloid culture has worked to not only normalize but prioritize the use of ART for infertile individuals to conceive. The continued exposure of mothers with multiples through tabloid media has made this mothering practice less obscure and more acceptable. Yet there are consequences to this newfound acceptance of conceiving and mothering multiples in the infertility community.

More feminist interventions are needed in the infertile community to displace this reliance on fixing infertility through cultural ideologies that privilege securing a family and fulfilling dreams of becoming a mother. Specifically, what is lost in the tabloid culture of mothers of multiples is the real health risk involved in conceiving and birthing multiples. While infertile couples often consider the news of conceiving multiples as a blessing, such a rhetoric that privileges nuclear conceptions of the biological family and the "natural" desire for the female partner to become a mother fails to account for the risk involved in ART. Feminist intervention to disrupt biopower's alliance with patriarchal constructions of motherhood is needed to begin asking critical questions within the infertility community. For example, how does the decision to receive fertility treatments affect gendered and cultural expectations of mothering? How can infertile women (re)conceive cultural practices of mothering? Women— and men—who cannot have children are still in position to mother individuals through a variety of practices and experiences. While this may not appear and function similarly to biological practices of mothering, there is need to consider how practices of mothering extend themselves to situations beyond that of the nuclear family. Doing so will begin to disrupt the relationship between ART and biopower, which fails to provide alternative options to the experience of infertility, such as the decision to live childfree or to adopt. As tabloid culture continues to instantiate itself into our lives, new versions of uncanny mothering practices must emerge to begin to make visible what is often assumed to be obscure in motherhood. Layne has cautioned against the publicity of the uncanny. While this publicity does in fact bring more awareness, Layne believes it often reinforces rather than changes social taboos. Layne's caution against the tabloidization warns that such publicity does little to change social taboos. While this may be true, I argue that the publicity does much for the particular community the tabloidization represents. In the case of Suleman, Gosselin and Gardner, all three have spoken in some regards to their experiences with infertility. As a topic often invisible to the public, publicity about the experiences of infertility begin to erode the stigmatization and silencing commonly felt by those suffering with it. The frequent belief that infertility can only be resolved through having a family (especially a biological family via fertility treatments) exposes the need for more feminist critiques of infertility. These critiques begin to reposition these assumed understandings and to disrupt biopower's normalizing and patriarchal control over the female body. Making visible even uncanny mothering practices begins then to ask critical questions about how cultural attitudes of motherhood construct uncanny identities. These are questions that must continue to be explored as ART enables new possibilities for embryonic motherhood.

NOTES

[1] By "Western," I am referring to those who live in the "Westernized" developed world as opposed to Eastern cultural practices and/or developing world cultural practices.

WORKS CITED

Biressi, Anita, and Heather Nunn. *The Tabloid Culture Reader.* Maidenhead: McGraw-Hill/Open University Press, 2008. Print.
Britt, Elizabeth C. "Medical Insurance as Bio-Power: Law and the Normalization of (In)fertility." *Body Talk: Rhetoric, Technol-*

ogy, Reproduction. Eds. Mary M. Lay, Laura J. Gurak, Clare Gravon, and Cynthia Myntti. Madison, Wisconsin: University of Wisconsin Press, 2000. 207-225. Print.

Celizic, Mike. "Everything I Do Revolves around My Children." *today.com*. NBC News, 2013. Web. 26 Oct. 2014

Centers for Disease Control and Prevention (CDC). "FastStats: Infertility." CDC, 30 May 2013. Web. 13 Nov. 2014.

Centers for Disease Control and Prevention. "Reproduction Health: Infertitlity FAQs." CDC, 30 May 2013. Web. 13. Nov. 2014.

Diepenbrock, Chloe. "God Willed It! Gynecology at the Checkout Stand: Reproductive Technology in the Women's Service Magazine, 1977-1996." *Body Talk: Rhetoric, Technology, Reproduction*. Eds. Mary M. Lay, Laura J. Gurak, Clare Gravon, and Cynthia Myntti. Madison, Wisconsin: University of Wisconsin Press, 2000. 98-124. Print.

Foucault, Michel. *The History of Sexuality, Volume I: An Introduction*. New York: Random House, 1990. Print.

Freud, Sigmund. *The Uncanny*. 1919. New York: Penguin Books, 2003. Print.

Greil, Arthur. "Infertile Bodies: Medicalization, Metaphor, and Agency." *Infertility Around the Globe: New Thinking on Childlessness, Gender, and Reproductive Technologies*. Eds. Marcia C. Inhorn and Frank Van Balen. Berkely: University of California Press, 2002. 101-118. Print.

Greil, Arthur, K. Slauson-Blevins, and J. McQuillan. "The Experience of Infertility: a Review of Recent Literature." *Sociology of Health & Illness* 32.1 (2010): 140-162. Print.

Kulkarni, A. D., D. J. Jamieson, H. W. J. Jones, D. M. Kissin, M. F. Gallo, M. Macaluso, and E. Y. Adashi. "Fertility Treatments and Multiple Births in the United States." *The New England Journal of Medicine* 369.23 (2013): 2218-2225. Print.

Lay, Mary M., Laura J. Gurak, Clare Gravon, and Cynthia Myntti. *Body Talk: Rhetoric, Technology, Reproduction*. Madison, Wisconsin: University of Wisconsin Press, 2000. Print.

Layne, Linda L. "Spectacular Loss: The Public Private Lives of the Santorums and Duggars at the Intersection of Politics, Religion and Tabloid culture." *Motherhood, Markets and Consumption: The Making of Mothers in Contemporary Western Cultures*. Ed.

Stephanie O'Donohoe. New York: Routledge, 2014. 222-236. Print.

Mamo, Laura. *Queering Reproduction: Achieving Pregnancy in the Age of Technoscience*. Durham, NC: Duke University Press, 2007. Print.

Marsh, Margaret S. and Wanda Ronner. *The Empty Cradle: Infertility in America from Colonial Times to the Present*. Baltimore: Johns Hopkins University Press, 1996. Print.

Murray, S. R. and J. E. Norman. "Multiple Pregnancies Following Assisted Reproductive Technologies—a Happy Consequence or Double Trouble?" *Seminars in Fetal & Neonatal Medicine* 19.4 (2014): 222-227. Print.

O'Reilly, Andrea. "Introduction." *The 21st Century Motherhood Movement: Mothers Speak Out on Why We Need to Change the World and How to Do It*. By O'Reilly. Toronto: Demeter Press, 2010. 1-20. Print.

Ornebring, Henrik and Anna Maria Jonsson. "Tabloid Journalism and the Public Sphere: A Historical Perspective on Tabloid Journalism." *The Tabloid Culture Reader*. Eds. Anita Biressi and Heather Nunn. Maidenhead, UK: McGraw-Hill/Open University Press, 2008. 23-33. Print.

Pawlowski, A. "After Eight Years of Infertility, Parents' Shocked Reactions to Quadruplet Pregnancy Go Viral." *today.com*. NBC News, 16 Oct. 2014. Web. 26 Oct. 2014

Pawlowski, A. "Gosselin Girls go Silent on Whether They're Doing Okay, Let Mom Kate Do the Talking." *today.com*. NBC News, 16 Jan. 2014. Web.

Reddy, Sumathi. "Fertility Study Warns of Risks from Multiple Births: Expert Counter Notion that Having Twins Is a Blessing." *Wall Street Journal*. 28 April 2014. Print.

Resolve: The National Infertility Association. "Fast Facts About Infertility." Resolve: The National Infertility Association, 19 Apr. 2015. Web. 27 Oct. 2014

Samakow, Jessica. "Mom Whose Reaction To Her Ultrasound Went Viral Gives Birth To Quadruplets." *Huffington Post*, 29 Dec. 2014. Web. 27 Oct. 2014

Sandelowski, Margarete J. "Failures of Volition: Female Agency and Infertility in Historical Perspective." *Signs: Journal of Women in Culture and Society* 15.3 (1990): 475-499. Print.

Sandelowski, Margarete J. and Sheryl de Lacey. "The Uses of a 'Disease': Infertility as Rhetorical Vehicle." *Infertility Around the Globe: New Thinking on Childlessness, Gender, and Reproductive Technologies.* Eds. M. Inhorn and F. van Balen. Berkeley: University of California Press. 33-51. Print.

Shivas, Tricha, and Sonya Charles. "Behind Bars or Up on a Pedestal: Motherhood and Fetal Harm." *Women and Children First: Feminism, Rhetoric, and Public Policy.* Eds. Sharon M. Meagher and Patrice DiQuinzio. Albany: State University of New York Press, 2005. 183-204. Print.

Closing

KATHY MANTAS

Besides being a mother of a daughter who is a lone twin and a daughter to a mother who is a twin, I am also a resident of North Bay, Ontario, in Canada. This northern city is where the Dionne Quints Museum, or original home in which the Dionne quintuplets were born, is currently located. The Dionne quintuplets, however, were born in the nearby town of Corbeil. Their home was moved from Corbeil to Callander in 1960, then from Callander to North Bay in 1985 (*Fact Sheet* 1).

The Dionne quintuplets were born two months premature to Elzire and Oliva on May 28, 1934.[1] The order of birth for the

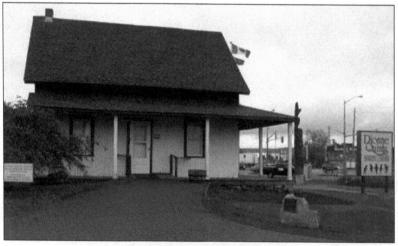

View of the Dionne Quints Home. October. 2015.
Kathy Mantas, photographer.

girls, by name, was: Yvonne, Annette, Cecile, Emilie, and Marie. They were born during the Great Depression and became world famous almost overnight. Francoise Noel states, "The chances of a natural identical quintuplet birth are one in 57 million. Small wonder that the vast majority saw the birth of the Dionne quintuplets as a miracle" (142). As far as we know, they were—and still are to this day—the first naturally conceived identical quintuplets to live to adulthood.

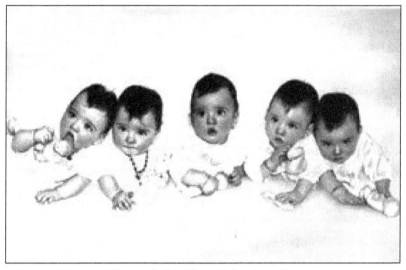

Photograph of the Dionne Quintuplets, 1934.
Dionne Quints Museum collection with the express permission of A. Dionne & C. Dionne

Although I have been living in North Bay since 2007, I did not visit the museum until this past summer (2015). I took a detour to the museum one day while I was out running some errands. It was a sunny weekday in July and, to my surprise, I realized that I was not the only visitor at the Dionne Quints Museum on this day; there were several others there as well. During my visit, I saw many artifacts, and read several stories. I even saw a short black and white film portraying the daily lives of the infant girls while they were in the care of the well-known doctor A R. Dafoe. As well, I spoke extensively with my tour guide—who focused on the history, context of the time, and dissipating falsehoods—about what I was viewing, and I took a number of pictures. In my efforts

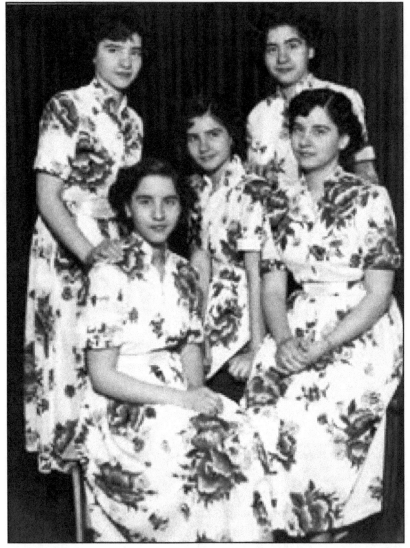

Photograph of the Dionne Quintuplets, 1951.
Dionne Quints Museum collection with the express permission of A. Dionne & C. Dionne

to gain a deeper understanding of the events, I even spoke with the museum director at length. She shared what she knew in a respectful and sensitive manner and encouraged me to do more research by providing me with a book list.

During the Great Depression, "almost three million people visited the Dionne quintuplets between 1934 and 1943, from their birth

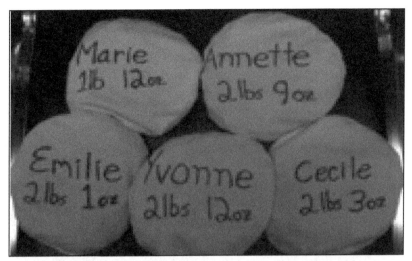

View of Bean-Bags with the Names of the Girls and their Weight at Birth
(Artifacts Created by Museum Staff), July 2015. Kathy Mantas, photographer.

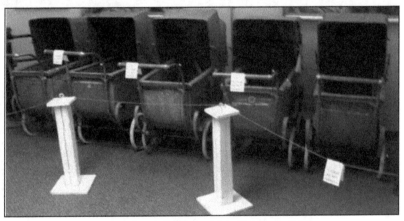

View of Dionne Quintuplets' Baby Carriages, 1934
(Museum Artifacts) July 2015. Kathy Mantas, photographer

to the age of nine—the period during which they were under the control of the Ontario government and on display for visitors to Quintland" (Noel 161). The Ontario government built Quintland, an observation playground, and when the Dionne quintuplets were two years of age, the public could watch them twice a day for thirty minutes (*A Brief History of the Dionne Quintuplets* 1). Fame, though, brings other complexities with it and so it did for the Dionne family, including the girls. As published in a local paper, "the Dionne Quints Museum is a collection of relics of a less-than-flattering chapter in the history of Ontario" (Young 3). [2]

But as my tour guide, the museum director, and the texts that I have consulted thus far, suggested, it is not easy to know the real story in this situation, as it is a multifaceted one. I left the museum, therefore, having gained some insight into this complex narrative, as this is reportedly the main purpose of the *Dionne Quints Museum*. I also left feeling both disturbed and provoked.

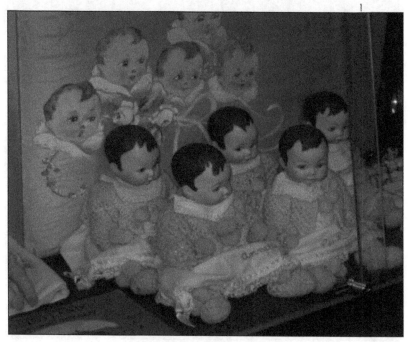

View of Dionne Quintuplet Dolls
(Museum Artifacts), July 2015. Kathy Mantas, photographer

During this visit, I was reminded again that we, as a society, have always been and continue to be intrigued by twins, triplets, and other higher order multiple births. Additionally, this confirmed for me once more that there is so much more that needs to be done with respect to attending to some of the disparities in our literature and experience on the topic of mothering multiples.

It is my hope that this collection of creative, scholarly, and blended essays that *are alike and not alike,* and which I have endeavoured to portray in a more fluid manner than in designated sections, has deepened our knowledge base of the many points of view through which the subject of mothering multiples can be contemplated. This volume has emphasized, for example, that mothering multiples entails many realities, simultaneously experienced: feeding and mothering twins, one of whom has special needs; breastfeeding twins; co-mothering twins; mothering twin girls, twin boys, and a twin girl and boy; mothering twins and older and/or younger siblings; mothering a lone twin after losing the other twin and experiencing the loss of both twins while mothering older siblings.

Moreover, by exposing, challenging, and providing insight into some of the complexities and possibilities inherent in mothering multiples, this collection—which does not put forth a singular "expert" voice but instead weaves together multiple voices from a wide range of disciplines and cultural perspectives—has attempted to broaden our understandings of the experience of mothering multiples. Some of the issues covered included the following: prematurity; high-risk pregnancy; affordable child-care; hostile environments (hospitals, fertility clinics and mothering environments); sexualization of breastfeeding; identity (of a mother of multiples and twin and/or multiple); community responsibility, support, and care; inadequate social supports; culture; trials and tribulations of daily life and living; infertility; assisted reproductive technologies (ART); queer reproduction; homonormative privilege; single mothers; social constructions of good mothering; maternal essentialism; and tabloid culture.

Furthermore, it is my wish that this volume not only has provided some insight into the complexities and possibilities but has also offered hope, raised questions, identified areas for further exploration, and contributed to ongoing discussions on the *fullness* of the experience—both complex and wondrous—of mothering multiples.

I would like to close this collection by sharing with you one of the images that stayed with me, and continues to preoccupy me, from my initial visit to the *Dionne Quints Museum*; it is the image of the commemorative stone located in front of the entrance to the original log house where Yvonne, Annette, Cecile, Emilie, and Marie were born. It honours the visit of Annette, Cecile, and Yvonne (the three surviving sisters) to the museum on May 23,

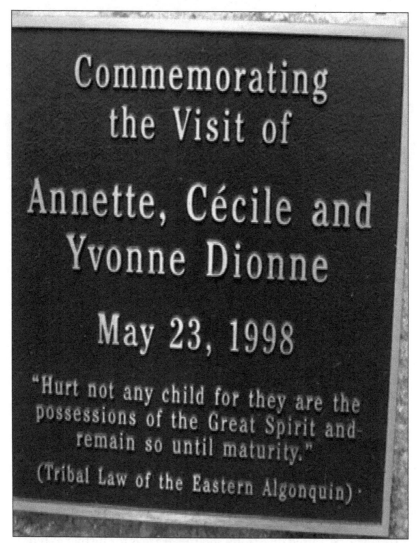

Commemorative Stone
July 2015. Kathy Mantas, photographer.

1998. I share it with you here as a way to encourage us to continue this worthy discussion and to leave us with something further to ponder regarding mothering multiples. More importantly, I share the image as a way of reminding us to proceed with care, compassion, respect, and sensitivity to multiples, multiple birth individuals, and their families in our efforts to gain and expand our knowledge on the experiences of mothering multiples.

NOTES

[1]May 28th, the birthdate of the Dionne quintuplets, has been proclaimed *National Multiple Births Awareness Day*. This initiative was started in 2005 by Multiple Births Canada (MBC), a non-profit organization that raises awareness about the various challenges and concerns faced by multiple birth individuals and their families. [2]"The Dionne quintuplets were removed from the Dionne home when they were almost four months old. They were moved to the Dafoe hospital (the nursery), where the government of Ontario took over the girls' names and they became Wards of the King. Nurses were hired on full time to give the infants the round-the-clock care that they needed" (*A Brief History of the Dionne Quintuplets* 1). The Ontario government made the Dionne quintuplets wards of the state when their father decided "to display the babies at the Chicago World Fair in an attempt to financially support his five premature infants (Noel 142-143) and his older children. The Dionne quintuplets were reunited with their family, their parents, and additional eight siblings, when they were nine years of age.

WORKS CITED

Dionne Quintuplets Museum. *A Brief History of the Dionne Quintuplets*. North Bay, ON: Dionne Quintuplets Museum, 2011. Print.

Dionne Quintuplets Museum. *Fact Sheet*. North Bay, ON: Dionne Quintuplets Museum, 2011. Print

Noel, Francoise. *Nipissing: Historic Waterway, Wilderness Playground*. Toronto: Dundurn, 2015. Print.

Young, Gord. "Fate of Dionne Museum in Limbo." *The Nugget (Community Voices)* 24 Sept. 2015, North Bay: 3. Print.

About the Contributors

Kirsten Eve Beachy is an assistant professor of English at Eastern Mennonite University in Harrisonburg, Virginia. She co-chaired a bi-national conference, Mennonites Writing VI: Solos and Harmonies, and is the editor of an anthology of Mennonite literature. Her short stories and creative non-fiction have appeared in journals such as *Shenandoah, Tusculum Review, Relief, The Cresset, Rhubarb, Spittoon, The Norton Anthology of Hint Fiction,* and Demeter Press's *Mennonite Mothering.*

Christie E. Bolch, MBBS (Hons), PhD, FRACP is an Australian paediatrician and mother of three, including identical twin boys born at thirty-two weeks. Her doctoral thesis regarding quality of life and psychological well-being of mothers of multiple birth children was completed in 2013. She is leading a study at the Murdoch Children's Research Institute, Melbourne, Australia, into developmental outcomes for survivors of twin-to-twin transfusion syndrome managed with laser therapy.

Cathy Deschenes is a mother of five: Daniel, twenty-one; Joshua, eighteen; Emily, thirteen; and Jordan and Katie, twins that passed away in November 2001. Cathy married her high school sweetheart, Joel, twenty-two years ago. She worked as a doula for fifteen years, assisting couples during their pregnancies, labour, and postpartum period. She has presented to healthcare professionals in Ottawa and in Las Vegas about the effects of multiple birth loss.

Jane R. Fisher, professor, BSc (Hons), PhD, MAPS, is director of the Jean Hailes Research Unit at Monash University, Melbourne, Australia, and is an academic clinical and health psychologist with long-standing interests in the social determinants of health. Her research has focused on gender-based risks to women's mental health and psychological functioning, in particular related to fertility, conception, pregnancy, and the perinatal period.

Lynda P. Haddon is a mother a four daughters, including dizygotic (fraternal) twins, and a multiple birth educator, providing support for over thirty-three years to parents and grandparents of multiples. She has taught and counselled over one thousand families attending her multiple birth prenatal classes and offers a DVD for parents not able to attend classes. Furthermore, she created and manages a fulsome educational website (www.jumelle.ca) brimming with information for both parents and health care professionals as well as an app from iTunes (Jumelle) so sleep-deprived parents can accurately record, among other things, which baby did what, when, and for how long. She is a frequent contributor on the subject of multiple births in the media and the community

Terri Hawkes has worked extensively across Canada and the U.S. as an actor, director, and writer in theatre, film, and television. She holds an Honours MFA in theatre, film, and television (UCLA), an MA in gender, feminist, and women's studies (York University), and is pursuing a PhD with a research focus on women in the arts. Publications include the anthologies *Performing Motherhood* (co-editor, Demeter 2014), and *Screening Motherhood* (contributor, Demeter 2016). She co-helmed two upcoming short documentaries, *Fourteen* and *Dr. Do*, and is currently writing a full-length play, *Mother Knows Breast*, adding to maternal herstories in film and theatre. Ms. Hawkes, with her teenagers, Alexa and Jake, co-founded *art4you*, an organization mentoring youth in the arts. art4you.ca; Twitter: @Terri_Hawkes; Facebook: http//on.fb.me/1HUEWQX

Jessica Jennrich has three children and lives in Grand Rapids, Michigan with her wife. She is the director of the Women's Center at Grand Valley State University. Her essays have appeared in

Paradigm Magazine and, most recently, her scholarly work has been published in the *Journal of Progressive Policy and Practice.*

Suzanne Kamata is an American lecturer at Tokushima University in Japan. She is the author of three novels, including *Losing Kei,* and editor of three anthologies, including *Love You to Pieces: Creative Writers on Raising a Child with Special Needs.* She has received numerous awards, including a grant from the Sustainable Arts Foundation, the SCBWI Magazine Merit Award for Fiction, and five Pushcart Prize nominations.

Jennifer Kelland completed her PhD in educational policy studies at University of Alberta (2011). While her research focuses on women learning online, as a mother of multiples, she is also interested in exploring issues related to being pregnant with and/or parenting multiples from educational and feminist perspectives. She also volunteers as the research coordinator for Multiple Births Canada (MBC).

Kathy Mantas is an associate professor of education at Nipissing University in North Bay, Ontario, Canada. Her research interests include ongoing teacher development, teacher knowledge and identity, adult education, arts education, artful and creative forms of inquiry, creativity in teaching-learning contexts and in women educators, holistic and wellness education, women's health issues, and motherhood and mothering studies.

Mangalika Sriyani Meewalaarachchi is from Sri Lanka and currently lives in Norway. She obtained her PhD in 2009 in Japan at Nagoya University, and her MBA (2000) and BSc in Agriculture (1998) in Sri Lanka. Presently, Mangalika is affiliated with the Meijo Asian Research Center at Meijo University in Japan. She has more than 20 publications in the fields of economics and social anthropology, and she also works as an artist/commercial designer, having received many awards for creative work including the Bergen Prize-Stipend in Norway in 2013.

Maria Novotny is a PhD student in rhetoric and writing at

Michigan State University, studying the medicalized discourse of infertility. Her research focuses on the intersections of rhetorical studies and medical humanities. Much of her scholarship requires collaboration with the infertility community to better assist medical professionals and legislators to understand the patient perspective of infertility. It is hoped that her research will foster greater public education about challenges individuals face when experiencing infertility.

Abigail Palko is the associate director of the Gender Studies Program at the University of Notre Dame, with affiliations with Africana Studies and Irish Studies. Her research focuses on representations of mothering practices in contemporary anglophone literature and society, especially contestations of motherhood as institution and questionings of heteronormative sexuality. In addition to practicing feminist mothering in her daily life with her partner and daughter, she is the 2013-2015 co-chair of NWSA's Feminist Mothering Caucus.

Rosemary Ricciardelli is an assistant professor in the Department of Sociology at Memorial University of Newfoundland. Her research interests include evolving conceptualizations of masculinity and experiences and issues within different facets of the criminal justice system. Yet, as a mother of multiples, her secondary interests are embedded in the institutional, personal, and social challenges surrounding parenting or birthing multiples.

Leslie Robertson is a lawyer by training and formerly of the feminist law firm Galldin Roberston where she worked primarily with low-income women, trans folk and non-traditional families. She She sits on the boards of the Ten Oaks Project and the Groundswell Community Justice Trust Fund.

Bonnie L. Schultz is a mother of four amazing adult daughters including monozygotic girls (identical twins). She is also an artist and avid quilter with long-standing interests in the arts, multiple births, and photography. Her *"BooLou Collection"* includes a limited-edition line of inspirational/positive affirmation photo cards, designed specifically for women. Bonnie has dedicated over thirty years to Multiple Births Canada (MBC), working with its founder to build its foundation, and acting as a consultant and contributor on the subject of multiple births via their website and publications. As well, she served as the Multiple Births Canada president for four years and business services manager for five years. Bonnie is likewise a fundraiser for a variety of causes. She is currently focusing on new creative endeavours in her ranch studio, world travel, and being a Gran to her three delightful granddaughters.

Celeste Snowber, PhD, is a dancer, poet, and educator who is an associate professor in the Faculty of Education at Simon Fraser University. Author of many essays and poems, books include *Embodied Prayer* and she is co-author of *Landscapes in Aesthetic Education*. Her last full-length performance was entitled, "Woman Giving Birth to a Red Pepper." Celeste is a mother of three amazing adult sons and her website is www.celestesnowber.com and her blog is at www.bodypsalms.com.

Erica Stonestreet is the mother of a singleton boy and twin girls. She is also a philosopher at the College of St. Benedict and St. John's University in Minnesota. Her philosophical work explores the moral significance of *who we are*, centring on love's role in building and shaping our identities.

Victoria Team, MD, MPH, DrPH, is a research fellow in the School of Social Sciences, Monash University. Her research interests are in the area of women's health. Her publications focus on body image, caregiving, disability, reproductive screening, and breastfeeding. She was trained as a general practitioner in eastern Ukraine and then practiced in Ethiopia for over ten years. Pot painting is her hobby.

Kathryn Trevenen is an associate professor at The Institute of Feminist and Gender Studies and The School of Political Studies at the University of Ottawa. Her teaching, research, and activism focus on queer cultures and queer theory; the intersections between feminist, trans and disability studies; and hip hop studies.